FATIGUE RECOVERY

The Ultimate Guide on Everything You Need to Know About the Causes

(Adrenal Fatigue and How to Reset Your Diet and Your Life)

Tracey Smith

Published by Andrew Zen

Tracey Smith

Fatigue Recovery: The Ultimate Guide on Everything You Need to Know About the Causes (Adrenal Fatigue and How to Reset Your Diet and Your Life)

ISBN 978-1-77485-191-3

Legal & Disclaimer

The information contained in this book is not designed to replace or take the place of any form of medicine or professional medical advice. The information in this book has been provided for educational and entertainment purposes only.

The information contained in this book has been compiled from sources deemed reliable, and it is accurate to the best of the Author's knowledge; however, the Author cannot guarantee its accuracy and validity and cannot be held liable for any errors or omissions. Changes are periodically made to this book. You must consult your doctor or get professional medical advice before using any of the

Table of Contents

Introduction

But what percentage of people care for it with the respect it ought to be? How many can affirm that they take care of themselves with the kind of care mother gives her newly baby?

I know that you've come here to find solutions to your health problem. I'm guessing that you don't want is to hear "It's Your Fault!" Maybe that's what believe I'm about tell you, but that's not my intention.

In our current world when someone is sick, they have various choices. The most popular option is to go down the medical approach. An entire business and system has been designed around this specific idea which has become the norm in the world of business.

The entire system is based on satisfying a specific need that is present in every one of us. This is the need to find an "magic pill". We all want to believe that all the issues in our daily lives can be addressed swiftly, effortlessly and without pain through the use of a miracle cure.

The problem is that health problems are rarely easy to fix. The medicines available do not treat illness, but instead assist a person in dealing with painful and uncomfortable symptoms that point to the existence of a deeper issue behind the scenes.

The thing that this approach often fails to consider is to look into the root of the issue. People often believe that their health issues are the result from genetics or random accident or some mysterious virus.

In the same way Doctors are frustrated by patients who refuse to make even the smallest lifestyle modifications. Smokers receive lung transplants...and return to smoking cigarettes when they are released from the hospital. Doctors have likely seen this many times.

If you're searching for a magical pill the book won't provide you with it. If you're willing to accept the notion that health only comes through a healthy lifestyle, this book is packed with facts that can help you change your life for the better.

There isn't a cure that can be guaranteed and this should not be considered a substitute for any other treatment that you're undergoing. Rebuilding your health may be a lengthy process. If you consider it you're probably not sick at night, so why would you expect to be well in the night?

A new perspective must be taken on by the person seeking help. This is the most important understanding that it is the body which heals. The only thing you can accomplish is to provide our body with optimal conditions that will enable it to do the task it's always striving to complete.

The goal is to bring people back in the optimal health you can get into.

There is no guarantee regarding this venture, however as life is precious, it really is worth doing everything we can to enhance and restore our health.

You are likely to will experience amazing outcomes right away once you implement some of the concepts within this guide. Health and vitality are yours by birth so is it not time you took it on?

Chapter 1: Finding Mental Energy

Mental energy is low when physical energy isn't created. So, if already experiencing a slowdown then you'll be tired too. Your mind informs you that you're not well and aren't able to do anything. Mind power is very effective. It makes sense that the best source of the power of your mind is inside. It doesn't mean that you must force yourself to perform actions. It's about changing your mindset.

People who are exhausted often have less mental energy. They're exhausted. They focus their minds on the exhaustion, and consequently suffer more. To stop the cycle, you have to go into the state of relaxation. This isn't simple when you're feeling down about yourself. But, the exercise listed below can aid you.

Exercise to relax

Relaxation can help your mind recuperate its strength. If you can get your mind energized, you're already halfway to gaining energy to fight fatigue. It is likely that you aren't doing anything therefore, take advantage of this time to assist your mind to get into a positive mindset that will bring back the energy you require. Different religions across the world endorse the practice of meditation, but currently the most important thing to realize is that all over your body there are energy centers. They are discussed when you are treated with acupuncture, and is also believed to be a part of Hindus who call them chakras. If your energy points or regions are blocked, imbalance or illness is experienced. This is what you experience when you are tired. Therefore, during this initial practice, what we're trying to do is focusing on the energy and trying to make them work exactly as meant to.

Lay on your bed and put as small an amount of pillows as you can comfortably manage. Should your head be positioned back it means that you can breathe more easily. Put your arms at your sides, and ensure that the clothes you wear is comfortable and doesn't have any tension anywhere else as this can hinder your progress of relaxing.

Shut your eyes, and begin using your heels. Tensify your toes then feel the tension and then let them relax. The toes will begin to feel heavy. While doing this, try not to think of anything other than the part of your body that you're focusing on. Make sure that you don't let outside noise get into your head. If there is a television inside the house, switch off the TV before starting!

Use the same method for the calf, knee, the thigh, and so on upwards until you get to your chest. Work with your arms beginning from your hands all the way to your neck, shoulders and finally the various parts of the face as well as the head. After you've relaxed all the body parts your body, sit still for a few seconds and focus on the breath. Breathe through your nose and focus on the air entering your body. After exhaling, you will you can feel the air rising upwards from your lower abdomen. After your relaxing session be patient in getting back to your regular routine. Be careful not to jump up too fast since your body will be in a state of relaxation. You might be wondering if it helps to boost your energy levels but chances are you've been unrelaxing for a long period of time. Maybe you're not getting enough sleep, or what you do get could be erratic. This could be the cause of the fatigue too and we'll work on this further in our book.

If you are able to include an exercise routine once a day, it can help restore circulation to your body. Additionally, the meditation exercises that will be covered in the next chapter can also help as your posture is at fault for your fatigue as as anything else. The position you sit in during meditation can help correct this, and also assists in focusing your thoughts on the energy that flows between the mind and body, which is important in the search to get rid of your fatigue issues.

In the next chapter we will be discussing a variety of questions regarding your lifestyle, which can help you determine the source of your energy deficiency comes from. They will allow you to focus on areas where you are experiencing particular issues and are not the same for all. However, in each of them, you will have questions that are pertinent to you. You have to tackle these in order to restore the energy you lost quickly. Some are easy to understand, and others may require you to take on changes that you didn't consider as being problematic. Trust me when I say that this method was developed by a person who was suffering from fatigue and has been utilized by those suffering from a variety of ailments and always performs.

The practice of relaxing stops negative thoughts from flowing even for just a few minutes. Once you are used to adding this to your routine you'll be feeling mentally rejuvenated and by itself can help you gain mental strength which can help to motivate you to do something to increase your physical energy. The body and the mind are interconnected and if you're uneasy and are unable to be positive it is likely that you lack energy and will persist for a longer time. Therefore, to ensure your calm mind include your relaxation into the mid afternoon or the in the early evening to ensure that you don't clash with your post-food time. It is not advisable to lay down and unwind after eating. It is at this time that you're likely to experience it difficult to relax since your body is trying to improve the digestion process.

Chapter 2: Identify The Cause Of Exhaustion

If you feel tired easily and it is impacting other aspects of your life, take note one of the most important steps towards complete elimination of the issue and increasing your energy levels and vitality is to determine the root cause. Fatigue or exhaustion may be related to a particular illness. Therefore, in certain instances you might need to talk with your doctor or medical professional. Here are the most common reasons for exhaustion that are medical:

Depression

Depression doesn't just cause you to feel depressed and empty, but it will take away all your energy. It could cause you to get sleepy and eventually lead to fatigue. The correct treatment of the root causes of depression by seeking professional's assistance is the first step towards resolving the issue.

Diabetes

It is the body's inability to make the right (type I) or sufficient (typeII) insulin needed to ensure proper sugar levels. Although some types of diabetes are manageable by a healthy diet and regular exercising, more serious types will require medication or insulin. Unsteady blood sugar levels are one of the main causes of exhaustion and fatigue, and may cause permanent damage for your body. This is why it essential that your blood sugar levels are checked regularly by you and your doctor.

Chronic Fatigue Syndrome

If you are suffering from Chronic Fatigue Syndrome, you'll experience a chronic fatigue that can persist for months. The cause could be physical or mental but there isn't a particular test to identify CFS. Eliminating and treating other reasons for exhaustion like diabetes, bad sleep and nutritional habits could be the sole method of treatment.

Sleep Apnea

Sleep apnea can be described as a condition that causes incessant interruption and resumption of your breathing when you sleep. This is a pattern that causes a insomnia and an insufficient supply of oxygen in your body. People who suffer from this condition often feel exhausted when they go to bed than prior to, because of the absence of quality sleep. Treatment options are available with the help of a doctor and the use of a continuous-air pressure unit (CPAP) during sleep. It is suggested that those who suffer from sleep apnea consult an expert physician to tackle the issue efficiently.

5. Overwork

A lot of us have demanding jobs, which could leave us exhausted. Hobbies, work around the house, and even garden work can make us feel exhausted. Being on time, seeking help when working hard and taking breaks can aid in reducing exhaustion.

6.Toxic exposure

A variety of professions expose us to pollutants and toxins that make us feel tired or tired. Chemical chemicals, dust, chlorine and other chemicals will not just deplete our energy, but can also cause long-term harm to our bodies.

7. Chronic inflammation

Inflammation is among the most frequent causes of fatigue . It can be caused by injuries or burns, stress as well as a diet that is not optimal and numerous other factors. Identifying the source and treatment is vital because chronic inflammation could be the leading cause of permanent damage on joints, skin and various organs.

8. Nutritional deficiencies

One of the main reasons for fatigue and faticity is a poor nutrition. If you're pushed to the limit emotionally and physically, having the correct amount of fuel into your body is vital. Do you want your vehicle to go on long trips with no fuel or with the wrong type of fuel? No, but it is common for us to require our bodies to do exactly do that. It's been said many times, but a balanced diet with fresh fruits as well as lean meats and grains are essential to avoiding exhaustion. The consumption of excessive alcohol and tobacco is also one of the main causes of exhaustion.

9. Negative emotions

It can be difficult to be positive when negative emotions like guilt, anxiety and fear are your main thoughts. Negative emotions can drain your energy and make you be exhausted all the time. Finding the root of these feelings, and talking with a trusted friend or professional can assist in eliminating or reducing the negative emotions to help you feel more active.

To battle fatigue and exhaustion, it is essential to determine the root cause of your symptoms. So, you'll be able tackle these issues quickly. If you suffer from an ongoing illness it is suggested that you speak with your doctor. But, you'll learn ways to treat other causes that are not obvious in the following chapters in this book.

Chapter 3: Pain And The Body

If you cut yourself, blood leaks out, and there's the sharp pain that follows. If you suffer from migraines and you are suffering from a constant headache that is throbbing. If you're burned and suffering from pain, it is painful and unbearable. There are many scenarios in which an individual is subjected to the pain of. The pain can vary in intensity and frequency can be identified. The definition of pain however, is not in the realm of.

What is Pain?

Pain is a complicated stimulus. There is no precise definition of it since it's a completely subjective experience. It is the main reason that people seek medical treatment. It is a sign that something is not right or damaged. According to the International Association for the Study of Pain defines it as "an unpleasant sensory and emotional experience associated with actual or potential tissue damage or described in terms of such damage".

In reality it isn't always connected to biological processes. Medical care can detect as well as treat pain that is physical however, there's another type of pain that is difficult, if it is not even possible to treat with medicine means...emotional pain. What exactly is pain? Pain can be described as is much beyond neural transmission and transduction of sensory information. It's a complex mix of emotions, sensations experiences, culture, and the spirit.

How Does the Body React to Pain?

The process of nociception or pain perception is the process by which the sensation of pain is detected and transmitted into the brain's central nervous system at the point of origin. It's totally different contrasted with normal stimuli such as pressure, touch and temperature. If the stimulus is not painful the normal sensory receptors are the first to respond. If the stimulus is painful stimulus, the nociceptors are the first to activate.

This procedure consists of many steps:

Point of source and contact with the stimulus where the stimulus originates could be mechanical like cuts as well as pressures, abrasions or pressure. It may also be chemically induced like burns.

Reception is an action that occurs when the nerve end senses the stimulation.

Transmitting - Once nerve ends detect a stimuli, they transmit their signal into the central nervous system via the network of neurons.

Perception - This is the place where the brain receives the signals for further processing and then action.

If you have break your hand there's many aspects that affect your feeling of discomfort. The first is the mechanical stimulation of the object that has cut you. The cells in your body are damaged and the release of potassium. This is why you experience the sharp, intense pain at the time of injury. Then, Prostaglandins, Histamines and bradykinins produced by immune cells infiltrate the affected area in times of inflammation. This is when your body defends itself against the external stimulus. You may experience a dull ache or numbness in the affected area.

Nociceptor neuronal pathways are found through the peripheral nerves. Signals are transmitted by the free nerve endings in the layers of the skin. The signals are transmitted into the spine via the dorsal root. They connect with spinal cord's neurons segment as well as up to three or more segments beneath and above where the entry point is. This is the primary reason it can be difficult to determine the exact location of pain in the body, particularly when the problem is internal.

Secondary neurons transmit signals upwards via the spineothalamic pathway. The signal is transmitted from the spinothalamic tract towards the medulla (brain's system) and finally to the thalamus. It is the central relaying point in the brain. Certain neurons also transmit signals to the medulla's receptors that control physical behaviour.

After the signal has been processed in the brain certain signals will travel across the brain's motor cortex through the spinal cord, and finally on to the motor nerves. The impulses trigger muscles to contract, which causes you to remove your hands towards the target.

What are the Types of Pain?

There are many kinds of pain. Doctors and neuroscientists categorize pain into three categories:

Acute Pain is a kind of pain that's caused on the body. A body injury such as a burn or cut creates an intense discomfort in the area. It is a sign of injuries and triggers actions from the brain. It can be a slow process or rapidly. Based on the nature of injury and the severity of the injury the pain may last for as short as one or two minutes up to an entire year. Once the wound begins to heal, however, the acute pain is gone.

Chronic Pain - It's an ongoing type of pain. It doesn't need the body to be responsive like acute pain. Chronic pain persists, even after the trauma has repaired. It lasts for longer than 6 months. One example of chronic headache is migraine.

Malignant or cancerous pain A type of pain that is associated with cancerous tumors. It's often connected to chronic pain; however, cancer-related pain is more intense and covers a greater region. The reason for this is that tumors infiltrate healthy cells, which in turn affects nearby blood vessels and nerves.

Chapter 4: Causes Of Fatigue

There are many causes for fatigue. There are a variety of causes. Finding the root source of fatigue can be an extremely difficult task. Many aspects that are blamed for the occurrence of fatigue have to be scrutinized independently to determine the extent of impact they have on indicators of fatigue. This is due to the fact that these conditions can exist regardless of regardless of whether someone is suffering from tiredness or otherwise. This test can be useful in determining the on the cause is a specific factor in causing fatigue. But, it is important not to ignore certain factors and not pay attention to other factors. It is crucial to consider even those that appear to have no adverse effects on the overall health in the human body.

To understand the sources of fatigue, we'll begin by categorizing them into their categories, as follows:

Lifestyle Factors That Cause Fatigue:

These are the factors that affect the way you live. These are affected by lifestyle, habits, values moral standards, as well as the financial status. They are influenced by:

* Sleep deprivation.

A lack of sleep can cause fatigue. People tend to overlook this aspect. Don't undervalue the amount of time you are sleeping. You must get enough sleep to function at optimum levels. A typical person requires between 7 to 8 hours of sleep each day. If you live a full and hectic lifestyle sleeping is often the first thing that we lose. Chronic insomnia, specifically when you're sleeping but not getting enough sleep is a typical reason. Modifying your sleep schedule can assist. The surrounding environment demands a lot of sleep and the advantages when compared with those who sleep in a calm and comfortable surroundings.

* Anxiety and stress.

Being stressed or overly anxious can cause mental and physical fatigue. Stress can have a significant affect on the body's physical health and prolonged stress can cause adrenal fatigue, which causes you to feel exhausted and fatigued. Constantly under stress can lead to fatigue resulting from stress. The tasks that have the effect of exposing your brain to pressure should be planned in as to provide sufficient breaks. Furthermore, people who participate with intense or attention-demanding tasks should have plenty of time and an ideal space to rest and sleep. Simply put it's not advised to be working your brains without taking breaks.

* Insufficient exercise.

The employees whose jobs do not require movement are more prone to fatigue even if they don't do physical exercise. It is recommended to attend gym classes. Simple exercises, such as an occasional walk or run at a time are not so demanding than gym workouts and can yield similar outcomes when it comes to fighting fatigue. Regular exercise boosts endurance and energy levels. If you are tired, you might not feel the motivation to put your energy to exercising as you believe that you'll get worse fatigued, but that is not the reality. Actually, it decreases the chance of fatigue increasing further.

* Vitamin D insufficiency and poor diets.

Your body needs a nutritiously balanced diet to function at its best. Consuming too much sugar and wheat, and not eating enough fresh fruits as well as fiber and vegetables can lead to fatigue that is chronic.

A well-balanced diet is a good investment in your well-being. It is advised to drink sufficient quantities of fluids. Avoid drinks that contain large quantities of caffeine. It is also possible that fatigue is caused to a lack of iron in your diet or due to issues with absorption of iron.

* Work conditions.

The term "working environment" refers to the location where you will spend the majority of your time working. It doesn't necessarily mean your workplace, where you are spending the majority of your working day working in the field. Stressful workplaces can cause mental fatigue. Working long hours or being exhausted can create feelings of fatigue. Night work is the main cause of fatigue as the body is built to sleep at night. The central clock in the body is controlled by the brain, in combination with neurotransmitters that regulate alertness and the state of sleepiness.

* Reaction to certain medicines.

Certain prescriptions and medications available over the counter like antihistamines, cold and flu medication and beta blockers can trigger fatigue. Certain antidepressants can also cause insomnia that causes fatigue. Examine all negative effects of any medication when you are constantly worried about fatigue.

Fatigue could be a side effect from certain medications , such as the lithium salts and ciprofloxacin and lithium salts beta blockers chemotherapy, radiotherapy and other chemotherapy drugs.

Medical Factors That Cause Fatigue:

There are a variety of medical conditions could be the reason in causing or aggravating fatigue. An accurate diagnosis is crucial to determine whether a particular medical issue is the cause the cause of fatigue. It is common for fatigue symptoms to disappear after making the proper lifestyle adjustments. If symptoms continue to persist it is recommended to see your doctor. The most commonly cited symptoms of fatigue that are caused by medical conditions are:

Anemia is a condition that can occur when your body has a loss of blood or isn't equipped to supply the body with blood cells to replace those that die naturally. In other instances, it could be because the body is suffering from an issue that causes blood cells die before their normal lifespan of 120 days has expired. Anemia sufferers have a hemoglobin levels lower than normal. Hemoglobin is responsible for the transportation of oxygen into body cells. If the capacity of oxygen transport is decreased it means that less oxygen is delivered to the heart and the muscles. In turn, it is harder to carry out normal activities.

Sleep disorders that are currently prevalent, such as sleep apnea, narcolepsy, insomnia, or sleep apnea.

Sleep problems result in the body not getting the necessary rest that is required from sleeping.

Chronic pain.

Most often it is because tissues that are damaged, broken or infected. In these situations, it becomes hard for the tissues to create energy.

The amount of blood flowing through the body depends on the availability of water that is a large part of it. A lower blood volume translates into decreased oxygen supply to cells of the body which can lead to fatigue.

Allergies that can cause hay-fever, or asthma.

Asthma can cause oxygen levels to decrease, which in turn reduces the capacity of body cells to create energy. When cells are starved of oxygen, it is possible to feel tired.

Diseases That Feature Fatigue:

Chronic fatigue can be a sign of a variety of illnesses and conditions. The main categories of conditions that cause fatigue are:

* Fibromyalgia.

This type of fatigue is manifested by the fact that you wake up feeling more exhausted than when you went to bed. This is because of a sleeping too little and not getting enough restorative sleep.

The most common mental disorder is depression. Other disorders cause depression.

Depression is a result of an increase in the levels of enzymes that control the energy and mood levels. They also degrade neurotransmitters. The high levels of these enzymes decrease the amount of neurotransmitters. Patients are tired and fatigued.

* Abuse of drugs.

The effects of drug abuse can disrupt sleep, denying our bodies of the benefits by restorative, deep sleep. Additionally, drugs induce depression and anxiety which is associated with higher levels of the enzymes that cause moods. Depression cause fatigue as described above.

* Cancer.

Some cancers are linked to the growth of cytokines, which can cause fatigue in those suffering from fatigue. In other instances, fatigue may be caused by cancer , increasing the body's need for energy, the weakening of muscles or altering hormones of the body.

* Blood disorders

These variables alter the oxygen carrying capacity of blood vessels to body cells. Oxygen is utilized to synthesize energy within the cells of the body.

* Endocrine diseases

Hyperthyroidism and hypothyroidism.

The disease is manifested by the deficiency of thyroid hormone. The sufferers experience insomnia and experience difficulty sleeping. A friend of mine with hypothyroidism complains of bone-numbing fatigue all the time his thyroid levels are higher than normal due to the dosage he is taking. The reasons for fatigue resulting from these disorders are diverse.

* Diabetes mellitus.

The result is lower insulin levels. Insulin plays a role in lowering blood glucose levels. It helps regulate how much glucose is present found in the blood. The blood is eventually stocked with more glucose than is needed. Astonishingly, the excess glucose causes cells starve even amid the abundance since the cells are unable to absorb the glucose. Insulin is of paramount importance since it functions as the catalyst to allow the breakdown of glucose into energy. If insulin is not in sufficient supply, cells are unable to absorb the glucose, and they end up hungry. This situation should be considered in the future when we talk about excessive sugars in the diet later on in the book.

* Chronic fatigue syndrome (CFS).

We'll examine chronic fatigue more in depth later. It will be clear the connection between it and fatigue.

* Autoimmune illnesses

* Multiple Sclerosis.

Autoimmune disorders are defined by the body of a patient acting as if their tissues are not their own and producing a continuous immune reaction against itself, causing damage to tissues and cells involved in the production of energy.

* Poor diet or eating problems.

The cause is primarily with the lack of balance of nutrients in foods and diets which cause deficiencies in the energy synthesis. We will look at these when we finish the book.

* Neurological disorders

*Parkinson's Disease.

These conditions are responsible for the body's inability to withstand the muscle contraction force because the peripheral, central and autonomic nervous systems are affected.

* Physical injury.

Trauma is associated with lower salivary cortisol levels following awaking, compared to control subjects that show neuroendocrine dysfunction that is a symptom that is characteristic of the chronic fatigue syndrome. Trauma from physical causes also play part in the triggering of the fibromyalgia condition and, consequently, fatigue.

* Arthritis.

Cytokines in excess are produced by the bodies of people suffering from Rheumatoid arthritis. Cytokines can cause fatigue.

* Sleep deprivation.

The body doesn't get the deep restorative state that results in relaxation.

It is also crucial to differentiate the causes of physical fatigue and those that cause emotional fatigue. The factors that cause physical fatigue are the cause of mental fatigue, and vice the reverse. But, certain factors may result in both mental as well as physical fatigue.

Factors Responsible for Causing Physical Fatigue:

* Sleep deprivation.

* Physical condition is poor and inactivity.

* Obesity.

* Environmental reasons that can cause stress, like extreme temperatures and dealing with the traffic or long waiting times.

* The side effects of medicines that are available over-the-counter like antihistamines, prescription medications like blood pressure medication.

Causes of Emotional Fatigue:

* Work in a safe environment.

* A significant change in our lifestyle.

* Anxiety and depression.

* Try to hide your feelings from the world.

Causes of Fatigue in Sjogren's Syndrome:

* Joints and muscles get inflamed.

* Hyperventilation: a condition which causes one to breathe more quickly than usual.

Hyper viscosity is a condition where blood becomes thicker.

*Distal renal tubular acidosis (DRTA) The disease occurs when the kidneys fail to remove acid in a proper manner.

* Hypokalemia (muscle weakness).

* Thyroid disorders: This is an thyroid glands that are infected. The thyroid system regulates body temperature. If it is not functioning, low body temperatures lead to fatigue.

* Haemolysis: Sometimes caused due to the breakdown in red blood cell count.

Note: In the case of Sjogren's syndrome, the previously reasons are not the only cause of fatigue in these patients as they are often accompanied by one of the other factors that cause fatigue.

Chapter 5: Cfs Symptoms

The majority of CFS cases develop abruptly. It is usually a result of the flu-like illness. The majority of people get sick within a couple of months of intense stress. According to one Australian retrospective study it was discovered that a small percentage of those that were affected with non-viral or viral pathogens later meet the requirements for CFS. The conclusion of researchers is that post-infectious syndrome is an authentic illness model that could be utilized in the study of one possible pathophysiological cause for CFS. However, the precise frequency of the condition and the precise amount of stress and infection the development of CFS are not fully understood at present.

CDC Criteria

The most widely recognized and widely used diagnostic criteria for research and clinical use of CFS is that from CDC in the United States. The advice from CDC is based on the achievement of three requirements, according to the following:

1. A new or non-lifelong appearance of severe fatigue lasting at least six consecutive months. The symptoms of fatigue should not be a result of physical exertion, and not significantly relieved through rest, and is not caused by any other medical condition.

2. The fatigue should result in a substantial decrease in the normal levels of exercise.

3. At at least 4 of the symptoms have to be present and last for at minimum six months.

o Memory impairment and/or concentration problems

The malaise after exertion chronic and persistent fatigue and sickness that follows exertion regardless of the type, whether mental or physical

o Sleep that is not refreshing

o Myalgia (muscle pain)

O Arthralgia (multiple joints)

Headaches (in the form or in severity that has not been experienced by the person before)

A Recurring or frequent sore throat

Swollen and/or painful lymph nodes (axillary or cervical)

The CDC provides a range of additional symptoms that might be found in the CFS situation. These are:

* Feeling of a fogged state (brain fog)

• Trouble keeping an upright posture or balance issues dizziness, even fainting

* Allergic or sensitivity to foods, chemicals or medications, food items and odors.

* Irritable Bowel Syndrome - such as constipation, bloating, nausea, stomach pain or diarrhea

* Night sweats, chills, or chills

* Visual disturbances such as extreme sensitization towards light or pain in the eyes and blurring

* Mood issues such as mood swings, depression, panic attacks, irritability and anxiety

CFS has several of the symptoms listed above, along with a variety of other illnesses. The reason for this is that the presence of these symptoms may also be indicative of different illnesses. So the CDC advises that individuals who suffer from these symptoms talk to a physician to rule out other possible illnesses, including the following:

* Lyme disease

* Major depressive disorder

* Sleep disorders

* Abuse of alcohol or substances

* Hypothyroidism

* Diabetes

* Lupus

* Mononucleosis

* Chronic Hepatitis

* Multiple Sclerosis

* Other malignancies

Apart from the other medical illnesses the symptoms of CFS could be result of side effects from certain medication. It is therefore important to remember if you are taking medications and what medications is being taken.

It is important to note that the International Consensus Criteria does not need to wait for six months prior to making an diagnosis, as opposed to CDC's. Particularly, they state that this is due to the fact that there's no other illness criteria that delays an diagnosis until the patient's been suffering from the disease for at least six months.

Effects on Individual Functioning

There are many variations in the consequences of CFS on the performance that an individual. The results of these variations are extreme. Certain patients can live normal lives, and others end up in bed so and are unable to manage themselves. For the vast majority that are CFS sufferers, the capacity to engage in daily activities (family school, work, or work) is significantly reduced for a considerable period of time.

The severity of the symptoms and consequent disability is the same for females and males. A large number of patients experience intense chronic pain that can reach an uncontrollable level. There are numerous instances in which significant decrease in physical activity levels has been documented. In addition, reports reveal a decrease in the difficulty of the tasks. The impairments are like those seen in other medical conditions, such as late-stage AIDS as well as rheumatoid arthritis the end-stage renal condition, lupus as well as chronic obstructive pulmonary disease. The extent to the extent CFS affects a person's overall health and functional health is more than other serious ailments like congestive cardiac disease, MS as well as type II diabetes mellitus.

In many instances there will be periods of relapse and/or relief from the signs of CFS that make the treatment of the condition more challenging. If a person feels better for a short period of time, the person might over-exert themselves in their daily tasks. This can lead to an increase in intensity of their symptoms after they return.

The percentage of people who work for patients of CFS is also different. Around half of them are unable to work. For the remaining part of those who are able to work, two-thirds of them get only a limited amount of work due to their medical condition. Over 50% are receiving disability benefits or temporarily sick leave. Only 20% of them are full-time employees.

Cognitive Symptoms

The cognitive signs of CFS generally are related to attention, reaction times and memory impairments. The range of these deficits is of 0.5 and 1.0 standard deviations lower than normal or expected. This is enough to have an impact on everyday activities. There are impairments ranging from mild to significant, in basic and more complex processing of information as and functioning in working memory which continue for long periods of time. There is a clear correlation with the deficiencies experienced by patients. However, intelligence reasoning, language motor speed, as well as perception abilities don't appear to be significantly impaired in any way.

Chapter 6: Foods Used In Chinese Medicine

For thousands of years over the course of thousands of years, Traditional Chinese Medicine has been essential to treating holistically human bodies. TCM uses herbal remedies for treating illnesses and stop them from occurring. I am convinced that TCM is a very easy but effective method of keeping the body and mind healthy and well.

Over the years, I've observed many of my friends taking advantage of Traditional Chinese Medicine. Through various natural remedies the patients are able to treat numerous ailments, like headaches, indigestion and insomnia. Utilizing the correct foods to prevent and treat various ailments has been a staple in Chinese Medicine. The diverse foods used to cure ailments are listed below:

1. Vinegar - Vinegar can be described as an ingredient that is readily found in the

kitchen. Although vinegar is used as a powerful cleaning agent, it's an essential ingredient in many recipes. There are numerous varieties of vinegar such as dark or aromatic vinegar as well as balsamic vinegar and apple cider vinegar. Chinese utilize the dark vinegar for cooking. Chinese medicine is said to make use of vinegar to treat various ailments.

It is utilized for treating diarrhea. It is given to the patient to help prevent depletion of electrolytes as well as fluids. Vinegar is recommended to be given to the patient 3 times per day to help eliminate the condition.

It's effective in the cure of acne. Although it is able to clear acne, it can help prevent it. It is recommended to use vinegar on a regular basis in order prevent and treat acne.

Vinegar is a great way to lower blood fats, and to reduce cholesterol. This will assist you lose weight and keep your weight off.

It can help improve the digestion of an individual. Use vinegar frequently in your meals to speed your digestion.

2. Ginger Ginger is considered to be one of the main ingredients used in Chinese cooking. It is used in nearly each Chinese dish. The primary reason for doing it is not to enjoy the wonderful flavor of ginger but also to reap its health advantages. When winter is approaching ginger tea is a drink is a staple in my diet. It helps me fight off the flu and cold. It not only does great things to my health, but it tastes delicious as well.

The root of ginger is thought for its warming properties. It has been proven to aid digestion and increase your immune system. The root can also be utilized in tea as a flavoring agent.

It can be used to lessen cough and phlegm in people. Consume ginger in small amounts 4 times per day to eliminate cough and Phlegm.

It is given to women who are pregnant to fight morning sickness. Anyone who is prone to motion sickness should apply ginger before they travel.

An easy recipe that can ease the winter chills is ginger baths. Make sure you have warm water available and smash a good amount of ginger into it. Make use of this water for the basis for a foot bath. In the tub, soak your feet. This is sure to help to feel more comfortable.

Ginger is an excellent treatment for vomiting and nausea. You can take a small piece of ginger and take it in a slow, steady chewing motion to relieve nausea. You could also cut a tiny piece of ginger and place it on the belly button. It will instantly reduce your nausea and make you feel healthier.

Another intriguing use for ginger is to reduce hair fall. Cut a small amount of ginger and rub it the hairline or over the area where you've noticed excessive hair loss. You'll notice a decrease in the fall of hair.

3. Coix seeds - An excellent source of carbohydrates, coix seeds also are referred to for their tears of Job. It's not as readily accessible as cereal or oatmeal, but when you do locate it, you must be sure to go for it. It is believed to be superior to cereal and oatmeal. They are also known to have less quick acting carbohydrates, which makes the ideal option to replace your regular carbohydrate. The traditional method to cook the coix seeds for meals involves soaking seeds with water for approximately an hour before boiling the coix seeds in milk or soup similar to porridge. I enjoy porridge without milk as I love the small pieces that go into my mouth. The many uses for coix seeds can be described as the following:

They are believed to stop the development of cancer cells within the body, because of their anti-cancer properties.

They help reduce the amount of water retained within your body. This helps to control weight. I owe my consistent weight for many years to these wonderful coix seeds.

The seeds have been proven to decrease the chance of swelling joints. Utilize the seeds often to deal with the issue of swelling joints.

They aid the digestive system work efficiently. If you be prone to digestive problems then you must include seeds on a regular basis in your diet. I've seen a huge increase in the quality of my food since I started incorporating the seeds as part of my daily diet.

The tea made using coix seed powder Coix seeds is believed to smooth the skin and increase the appearance of youth.

4. Gouji berries - Rich in nutrients, gouji berries are renowned all over the world for being one of the best superfoods. It is widely found in the west and is also known

as Wolfberries. They are tiny in size and are often compared to red raisins. They are available in health shops. It is recommended to include gouji berries as a daily item in your diet due to their amazing health advantages. Many struggle to find the best way to incorporate them in their diet. There are a variety of ways in that you can consume these fruit. You can mix them into your smoothies and drinks of choice or incorporate them into salads. The berries can be utilized in soups, porridges stews, yogurt and soups. My friends often make tea with them. Simply add the berries to hot water and make tea as usual. The different uses for gouji berries can be described as the following:

The berries are believed to be extremely effective in eliminating constipation. They can also be used to delay the appearance of constipation when consumed regularly.

Gouji berries can be used to help prevent the development of conditions like diabetes. If you have an ancestral with a history of diabetes must take into consideration using gouji berries.

Gouji berries have been known to boost the immune system. If you consume them regularly and regularly, you'll see an improvement in your protection against many illnesses.

The berries have the ability to increase the quantity and quality of blood flowing through the human body. Other bodily fluids can also be positively affected by the fruit.

They are extremely useful to protect the liver of a human. Consume them frequently if you wish to have a strong liver for the rest of your life.

Chapter 7: Foods To Work Into Your Diet To Help

There are a variety of foods that you can incorporate into your diet to combat chronic fatigue, too. These are the food items that are easy to incorporate into your diet, and you'll discover recipes for each one that can help you manage your chronic fatigue without sacrificing taste.

Cacao powder is recommended for chronic fatigue due to its ability give you an energy boost while providing nourishment to your brain as well as your heart. It's beneficial to your overall health, and especially digestion health. It's well-known to help you through the day and it can be put to smoothies, or baked. But including it in your breakfast smoothie or snack is known to be the most effective.

Example Recipe: Cacao & Banana Blend

Ingredients:

1 Tablespoon Cacao Powder

2 Teaspoons Honey, Raw

2 Small Bananas, Sliced & Frozen

1 Cup Strawberries, Fresh

1/2 Cup Ice

1/2 Cup Almond Milk, Vanilla & Sweetened

Directions:

Simply put all the ingredients in the blender and blend until it is smooth. If needed, add more ice to make it more thick. It is also possible to add honey if you wish for it to be sweeter.

Kale as well as other deep greens is a great choice for those suffering with chronic fatigue. It's loaded with vitamins, minerals antioxidants, and minerals which will assist in keeping your body in top shape even if you're sleepy, tired or exhausted regularly. It could even help prevent anemia and are loaded with iron to aid your body.

Example Recipe: Kale & Shrimp Dish

It even has sweet potatoes in it which will aid in getting enough kale to your diet. You'll also see this can also be used in smoothies. It's an excellent sweet and savory meal which you can make every day and is perfect to eat for dinner or lunch. It's also easy to heat.

Ingredients:

2 Tablespoons Olive Oil, Extra Virgin

1/2 Teaspoon Red Pepper Flakes

1/2 Cup Onion, Diced Small

2 Cups Sweet Potatoes, Diced

2 Cups Shrimp, Fresh

3 Cups Kale, Chopped

1/4 Teaspoon Black Pepper, Ground

1/2 Teaspoon Sea Salt, Fine

3 Cloves Garlic, Minced

Directions:

Make use of a medium saucepan, and cook it over medium heat , while pouring into your extra-virgin olive oil. Add in the red pepper flakes as well as diced onions, and cook until the onions become soft and golden.

Incorporate the garlic and continue cook for another 30 seconds.

Include your sweet potatoes and cook for ten to fifteen minutes or until they are soft. You might need to add water to cook the potatoes.

You can then add the shrimp to cook until they are pink. This typically takes between two and four minutes.

Reduce the heat to low then add in the Kale, and stir until it's it is soft. Add salt and pepper and serve.

Blueberries are also a great fruit to include in your diet if you suffer with chronic fatigue. This is due to the fact that the chronic fatigue disorder can cause an increase in oxidative stress, which can be detrimental to your body and your appearance. Blueberries help to heal this damage, which is why you should include the fruit whenever you can. Blueberries are extremely antioxidant-rich.

Example Recipe: Banana & Blueberry Bread

This bread can be eaten all day long and is loaded with lots of antioxidants. The blueberries are delicious, even if you're using frozen blueberries. When baked into this bread, you'll contain enough blueberries to reduce the oxidative stress and is a great snack all day long.

Ingredients:

2 Cups Flour, All Purpose

1/2 Teaspoon Sea Salt, Fine

1 Cup White Sugar

1/2 Cup Butter, Softened

1 Teaspoon Baking Soda

2 Large Eggs

2 1/2 Teaspoons Vanilla Extract

2 Medium Ripe Banana, Mashed

1 Cup Blueberries, Fresh

Directions:

Begin by heating your oven to 350 degrees. then you can take three loaf pans and grease them with cooking oil to make them.

Use a medium-sized bowl for mixing your flour with salt as well as baking soda.

In a different bowl, mix sugar and butter, mixing it until it becomes soft and fluffy. Add an egg and then continue mixing with vanilla extract. It is then time to mix and mix into the banana before adding the flour mix.

Continue beating until they mix to form an even batter. after that, tart it to incorporate your blueberries.

Pour the batter into the loaf pans, then put them on the baking sheet. Cook for 30 to 35 minutes. The golden brown should appear at the top.

Lentils are a great source of plant-based protein and are abundant in minerals, which can help to fight fatigue-related effects. It will provide the energy boost you need and is perfect to include in curries, soups, and soups. If you're feeling tired it is important to look for food that can increase your energy level. You can bring soups in a thermos. So, it's a great option for lunch or even a meal.

Example Recipe: Spinach & Lentil Soup

This is a simple lentil and spinach soup and both spinach as being a dark green, as well as the lentils will assist you in fighting fatigue. If you add ginger, you've got an effective recipe for fighting fatigue which is guaranteed to ease your fatigue.

Ingredients:

3 Cups Water

5 Ounces Spinach

1 1/2 Teaspoons Cumin< Powder

1/2 Teaspoon Ginger, Grated

1 Teaspoon Smoked Paprika

1/4 Teaspoon Sea Salt, Fine

15 Ounces Diced Tomatoes

2 Cups Lentils, Dry

5 Cloves Garlic, Minced

3 Medium Carrots, Peeled & Chopped

1 Medium Onion, Diced

Directions:

Cut your carrot and onion first, then place it into a stockpot. It should be set to medium-high heat. You must cook for seven to eight minutes. Include your cumin, ginger, salt, paprika and garlic. Allow to cook for one minute, then add the broth, water, lentils, tomatoes and. Then, increase the heat and let it simmer.

Once it has reached a boil, reduce the heat, then cover. It should simmer for twenty five to 30 minutes. The lentils should be cooked. It is important to ensure that the spinach is well-chop.

Just before you're finished cooking, add some salt, and then spinach. Let them wilt and then serve.

Many oils can help reduce fatigue naturally for instance, coconut oil being just one of the most effective. A different one is olive oil and sesame oil. It is possible to cook with them, however you can incorporate into your recipes too. The reason is that they are an excellent fuel source for the body. They can also help improve blood pressure as well as your immunity. Yu can also make use of flaxseed oil. It can also help to reduce muscle and joint discomfort that may result from fatigue over time, and thus assists in relieving fatigue and the symptoms it causes.

Example Recipe: Blended Smoothie

The smoothie is refreshing mix which allows you to incorporate coconut oil easily. It is possible to use other oils too however coconut oil is the best blend and has an amazing flavor that you'll enjoy in this drink. You can even make use of coconut milk as well, which is believed for its ability to strengthen the muscles.

Ingredients:

1 Cup Coconut Milk

2 Teaspoons Honey, Raw

1/4 Cup Ice

1 Cup Strawberries, Fresh

1/2 Cup Mango Chunks, Frozen

3 Tablespoons Coconut Oil

Directions:

Blend all ingredients until the mixture is thick and smooth. Add as much or less ice required.

Salmon like any protein from animals is an excellent choice when you're trying to combat fatigue. The body requires protein to replenish energy and when you're tired, it's the first thing you require. It is essential to have energy to make it through your day. Salmon can supply it and is a fantastic food source for omega-3 fats, too.

Example Recipe: Lemon & Herb Salmon

This is the lemon and herb salmon recipe that is simple to prepare, and you can serve it with whatever side dishes you'd like. You can serve it in a meal or as a stand-alone lunch. Salmon is a nutritious fish that you can eat anytime you'd like.

Ingredients:

3 Ounces Butter

1 Teaspoon Fresh Dill, Chopped

4 Salmon Fillets, 5 Ounces Each

1/4 Teaspoon White Pepper, Ground

2 Cloves Garlic, Chopped

1 Tablespoon Parsley, Fresh & Chopped

2 Teaspoons lemon zest

1 Teaspoon Sea Salt, Coarse

Directions:

All the ingredients, minus that of the salmon may be put in a bowl, then placed in the microwave to soften. It should take between thirty and 45 minutes. Stir to ensure that the ingredients mix thoroughly.

Pick up your salmon fillets and set the fillets on top of a baking tray coated with parchment.

Use a pastry brush and apply the salmon to the butter mixture. It should be evenly spread across the surface.

The oven must be set at 400 degrees. Cook the salmon for ten to 12 minutes. The salmon must be cooked to perfection and should flake easily.

Beware of foods that can make you tired such as foods that contain excessive artificial ingredients or excessive sugars. You should choose food items that boost your energy naturally when fighting symptoms of chronic fatigue. Incorporating whole grains into your diet can help fight chronic fatigue. Eat these meals regularly throughout the day and you'll see that it aids in preparing your body for fighting fatigue, allowing you to be able to get throughout the working day.

Chapter 8: Developing A Healthier Mindset At The Workplace

As you are likely to spend most of your day working It is important to adopt a more positive mental attitude to work from. Being a positive person means working within your capabilities, striving for continuous improvement, creating pathways to relax, cultivating more positivity, and establishing an effective support system to assist you in dealing with the challenges you face.

To begin, put things from a different perspective. Consider your work as part of a larger picture which has to do with your own personal or professional objectives. If you see your work as a punishment, you create the appearance of a Sisyphean burden on yourself, which will only add your stress level. need to deal with all day long and every day out.

Signing up to the myth of perfection

One of the common pitfalls experienced by a lot of people and businesses is to believe in the notion of perfection. The "perfect" myth is counterproductive since at its simplest it requires you to define unrealistic and unreasonable expectations that are not met. When this is put within the context of the workplace it creates a work environment that is extremely difficult to manage, especially when every thing that's not "perfect" is automatically deemed as a failure. If all efforts and effort don't meet the ideal of perfection it is easy to become overwhelmed, if you don't completely demotivated and lose the determination to continue.

The secret is, obviously, to set expectations that rest on a realistic and practical basis. It is essential to be aware of your limitations and take advantage of opportunities to make the most of the resources you have, as you strive to constantly seek improvement. In this way, you will be able to sustain within your work without having to endure unnecessary stress.

One of the most important aspects to be aware of your limitations is the ability to say"no. If you're overwhelmed by projects that were essentially created because you kept saying yes to every one of them, you're in fact setting yourself up to be disappointed, anger and even failing. Be honest with yourself. If you don't see a possibility to do one more job to your existing inventory, then you must have the guts to reject the task. By doing this, you will avoid burning out and also saves your company from having to handle the consequences of a poorly-executed or incomplete task.

Awakening more positive energy

Create a positive outlook in your life by gaining lessons from your life and incorporating the same lessons into your everyday activities. Make sure you are constantly improving yourself by reflecting on your experiences in the past to improve your current situation. Are there strategies or techniques that have helped you deal an issue previously? Are you able to say that having a certain mindset towards a particular job in the past useful in alleviating stress and tension that you were under at the time?

It is also helpful to employ laughter from time to time to assist you in dealing with your current situation. Laughing can help lighten the mood of an anxious situation and helps you relax. Being too serious about things can cause a lot of pressure and stress that can eventually be a sting in the back. Have fun and relax. some enjoyment.

Finally, build an effective base of support. Be surrounded by your loved ones and family members to motivate you. You should surround yourself with people who inspire your best qualities and avoid people who are negative and a source of stress.

Chapter 9: The Adrenal Reset Power Boost Diet

As was mentioned earlier food is a major factor to the recovery of adrenal function. A variety of foods can be utilized to boost the health of your adrenal glands. They do more than give you a boost of energy and fill your appetite, but provide your energy levels to power your activities all day. There are many other ways that food choices can benefit you when trying to improve your health and well-being. However, first, you need to learn more about you can get from the Adrenal Reset Power Boost Diet is all about , and also what this diet could provide for you.

Definition

It's called the Adrenal Reset Power Boost Diet is a brand new diet developed by experts in wellness believing that adrenal fatigue could be a cause of fatigue, weakness as well as insomnia, depression and inability to concentrate, and a host of other signs. The plan is focused on eating foods that promote adrenal health and replenish energy levels in the adrenal glands. Here are some important information about this diet plan: Adrenal Reset Power Boost Diet:

Eliminating foods that tax your adrenal glands

Untreated and chronic stress can result in exhaustion of the adrenal glands. So it is sensible to limit any further stress on the glands. There are numerous ways in which the adrenal glands may be stressed when eating unhealthy food. Foods that are preservative-laden and artificial colors or flavors and other chemicals must be avoided at all costs. Also, any fruits and vegetables, grains or dairy products grown with pesticides, fertilizers, or fungicides must be avoid. Instead, search for foods that have an official "Organic" label.

The adrenal glands can also be more stressed when food items which trigger an allergic reaction are consumed. A food allergy could overwork the immune system and , consequently, strain the adrenal glands further. Someone who is suffering from an allergic reaction can suffer from hives, swelling, breathing difficulties or anxiety. All of these can cause the adrenal glands to become overworked and may cause more symptoms.

Consuming fresh healthy, natural, whole food items

Beware of preservatives, artificial flavours as well as dyes and other chemicals that are used in the processing of food and instead, eat organic and whole food. In doing this you give the adrenal glands room to recover.

Fresh and natural food items are healthier since they are freshly harvested from the fields. Natural foods are not contaminated with harmful toxins that could cause chronic diseases and, consequently, put more stress to the adrenal glands.

Selecting foods that are not processed

Avoiding foods containing hydrogenated oils

Making sure you are eating your meals at the right time

In between meals, eating several hours apart is a way to aid your body in digesting the food you consume and fully reap the benefits of the nutrients in these foods. Spacing your meals allows the body to fully digest food and more effectively absorb nutrients and process fiber. It also lessens stress upon the adrenal glands to make hormones necessary to regulate the metabolism of proteins, carbohydrates, and fat. Should the adrenal glands already tired, spacing meals makes sure that the gland isn't stressed to the point of exhaustion.

This is also true for instances when we don't take in food for a lengthy amount of time. The adrenal glands are in constant use to ensure that the body is performing its normal functions, and also release more adrenaline and cortisol when we are fasting. When blood sugar levels in the body drops during an extended period of food craving, the body gets stressed, which impacts your adrenal glands. It is therefore crucial to keep in mind:

1. The body requires energy to function properly even when asleep. Cortisol helps keep blood sugar levels steady between meals as well as at night. Thus, managing our meals to ensure we have enough energy to go to fall asleep is essential.

2. Healthy and timely small meals that are eaten at regular times throughout your day can ensure that energy is evenly distributed throughout the day.

3. The timing of our meals can help regulate cortisol levels through the day.

Cortisol regulates our sleep-wake cycles (called the circadian rhythm). Cortisol levels increase approximately 6 am, and then rise to peak around 8 am. The level fluctuates throughout the day and is at its lowest at night, particularly when we're asleep. Knowing this pattern can give us an idea of when to have larger portions and also when it is best to eat light meals.

4. The heavier meals should be consumed in the early morning hours in the morning, when cortisol levels are elevated to prevent pressing your adrenal glands. Foods that are lighter should be consumed during the latter hours of the day, when cortisol levels decrease.

5. In the course of the day, plan nutritious meals and snacks. For example eating fruits and vegetables that are fresh and healthy in the afternoon is more nutritious than eating processed foods or junk food. Healthy snacks can also make you feel fuller for longer, and help you avoid overeating.

Vital nutrients to support adrenal health

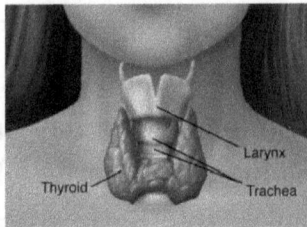

A significant portion of an Adrenal Reset Power Boost Diet plan is the utilization of minerals, vitamins and micronutrients. They are available in supplements that can be purchased at numerous health, grocery or drug stores with or without prescription. These nutrients are essential in restoring your endocrine system . They can improve the well-being that of your adrenal glands.

1. Control stress hormones using vitamin C, E and B complex. These vitamins help to improve the health of your immune system and aid in helping your body deal with stress each day.

2. Magnesium is a mineral that can be found in dark-green, leafy veggies as well as seeds, nuts and beans, whole grains as well as bananas, yoghurt and dark chocolate to only a handful of. Magnesium is useful in controlling the energy supply in your adrenal glands.

3. Calcium is present in milk, cheese seafood, yogurt, legumes as well as leafy greens and fruit. Calcium aids in managing stress and relaxes the body.

4. Trace minerals like manganese, selenium, zinc and iodine are essential to support the health of the adrenal glands and decrease stress.

Supplements will increase the amount of nutrients you can get from the foods you consume every day. It is not possible to get all the necessary nutrients and vitamins in the daily menu. Thus, taking nutritional supplements can assist.

Important:

If you have an illness that requires medical attention or are currently taking prescription medications it is recommended to consult your doctor prior to using any type of diet supplement. Any kind of over-the-counter supplement could lead to unsafe interactions, which is why it should be authorized or recommended by your physician.

Benefits

It is the Adrenal Reset Power Boost Diet is a brand new diet developed with the help of established nutritional data. It is said that, as the name implies it will help to reset the adrenal glands of your body, increase their performance, and help ensure that your adrenal glands are in good health and functioning to their maximum. It's also a diet that could provide the following advantages:

Improved metabolism

When stress levels are high then the adrenal glands release cortisol, which signals the body to increase to an increased condition of emergency. The body is compelled to defend itself against injury by heightened sensory. But, when your body experiences constant levels of stress and stress, the adrenal glands counter by constantly releasing an elevated levels of cortisol. In the end, this may weaken the glands.

Cortisol levels that are elevated can affect numerous metabolic functions within the body. This includes the natural functions of digestion and sleep as well as immune system functions in addition to the generation of different kinds of hormones.

The body's function is weakened through constant stress levels.

The Adrenal Reset Power Boost Diet Plan to Improve Metabolism:

1. Let the adrenal glands rest for a while. Through eating healthy, fresh, and natural foods that are easy to digest, your adrenal glands can relax and recover from stress.

2. Let the adrenal glands recover. Long-term exposure to stress wears the adrenal glands out. A diet made up of more nutritious food options lets the body get the most benefit from various nutrients, including minerals and vitamins. The intake of these nutrients can help to improve the health and wellbeing of your adrenal glands.

3. Let the adrenal glands rest by consuming food at a specific time. When following this kind regimen, meals intake is scheduled at specific times throughout the day, based on the natural fluctuation of cortisol levels. The result is less stress on glands.

Hashimoto's Disease

It is frequent for patients with Hashimoto's illness to also suffer from adrenal fatigue. Hashimoto's disease is a disorder where the immune system is able to attack the thyroid gland. The thyroid glands are situated at the neck's base under the larynx. The thyroid gland's job is the production of hormones which are required for numerous bodily actions.

When the thyroid gland gets inflamed following an attack by a virus, it is unable to function properly and causes the condition of hypothyroidism. These glands make less hormones due to the effects of inflammation. This may cause symptoms like fatigue as well as more sensitive to cold temperatures constipation, dry and pale facial skin, hoarse voices unanticipated weight growth, joint and muscle stiffness and pains, facial puffiness and heavy menstrual bleeding. Patients with Hashimoto's disease can also be suffering from stress and depression.

Adrenal Reset Power Boost Diet for Hashimoto's Disease

1. Reduce the stress to your thyroid gland. Consuming fresh, natural and unprocessed food can ease the workload on the gland when it comes to managing the

metabolism of the body. It will also be more able to digest food and transform it into energy that the body to utilize throughout the day.

2. Let the thyroid gland rest and recuperate. If the thyroid gland does not get being pushed to produce hormones that aid in the regulation of metabolism, it can be able to rest and recover.

3. Let thyroid hormone replacement drugs to function. Hormone replacement therapy (HRT) to treat Hashimoto's Disease functions by providing our body with hormonal substances that aid in the process of metabolism. When combined with a healthy food regimen, HRTs become more effective and can aid in helping the thyroid gland recuperate more quickly.

4. Give the body energy and nutrients your body requires. It is the Adrenal Reset Power Boost Diet ensures that your body

gets sufficient energy and nutrients to fuel the body for every day tasks.

Important:

If you are taking medications or hormonal replacement therapy for Hashimoto's Disease or other disorders affecting the endocrine system, you should consult your doctor prior to beginning any type of supplement or diet. Also, be aware that some doctors have been slow to recognize the issue that is Adrenal Fatigue.]

Sleep disorders

One of the long-term side effects associated with adrenal fatigue can be a lack of sleep. If the body is under perpetual stress levels, levels of cortisol are high , which can lead to a variety of sleep disorders like insomnia and disturbed sleep.

The Adrenal Reset Power Boost Diet Plan to Resolve Sleep Disorders

The ability to have an uninterrupted, restful evening sleep is essential in resetting your adrenal glands. The combination of several strategies will increase chance of getting the sleep which your adrenal glands require.

1. The adrenal glands to make cortisol levels slowly return to normal levels.

2. The adrenal glands are allowed to rest with a timed consumption can also lower the levels of cortisol. This can assist in returning body functions back to normal. In the end, you'll get free of sleeping disorders, and normal sleep-wake cycles are expected to return.

3. In taking in a healthy, rich in nutrients, the body benefits from the minerals and vitamins (such as magnesium, potassium and vitamin D, as well as melatonin) that regulate sleep.

4. When you eat nutritious, fresh and complete foods, your body can generate more energy throughout the day. Being

able to have a steady flow of energy throughout the day aids in regulating the cycles of wake and sleep. which can lead to better sleep at night which is the ideal time to unwind and fall asleep for the majority of people.

Important

A few sleep disorders or chronic insomnia could be due to illnesses that are underlying. If you've had a diagnosis of insomnia because of an illness that is underlying it is recommended to consult your physician prior to using any supplements or adhering to any diet regimen.

Hypoglycemia

Adrenal fatigue and stress could cause lower blood sugar or even hypoglycemia. Certain hormones that control blood sugar levels such as cortisol, norepinephrine, and epinep can be affected.

Stress is a signal to the body to be prepared for anything, which is why the body reacts with increasing the levels of blood sugar. If, for whatever reason, your body isn't able to cope with the needs from stress, then hypoglycemia, or unhealthy blood sugar swings can be observed.

When the levels of adrenal hormones are low because of the glands' inability to regulate for the loss, it becomes harder for your body keep the balance of sugar levels. People can feel irritable as well as weak, anxious and sleepy.

The body's natural process to regulate sugar levels is a complicated procedure - any condition can cause the condition of adrenal fatigue and hypoglycemia. Treatment to fix the imbalance might not suffice. The people who suffer from this condition should also take the proper diet to improve adrenal function, and eventually aid in resolving hypoglycemia.

The Adrenal Reset Power Boost Diet Plan for Hypoglycemia

1. Let the adrenal glands rest and rest and. Through eating natural, unprocessed and fresh foods the adrenal glands do not need to work as hard to make the hormones that help in the metabolic process. The adrenal glands are given the opportunity to rest and replenish themselves.

2. Healthy foods or food items which contain nutrients that enhance adrenal health could aid in improving the glands' hormone production, which results in improved performance and better absorption of nutrients.

3. Timing your food intake is crucial for those with hypoglycemia order to manage blood sugar levels and other signs of hypoglycemia. The key to a healthy diet is eating small , frequent meals throughout the day in order to benefit of the fluctuating levels of cortisol in the body.

4. Fresh and natural food intake helps to reduce the accumulation of toxins within the body, which increases the adrenal health. Toxins build up and can cause many health conditions that impact the body's ability to absorb sugar. Making a commitment to eating healthy and natural foods will lessen the chance of developing this condition and ultimately result in a healthy adrenal system.

Important:

The conditions of diabetes and hypoglycemia are treated with diet, medications and lifestyle modifications. If you've been diagnosed with diabetes, don't consume any kind of supplement or follow any diet or supplement without the approval of your physician. The hypoglycemia that you experience may be caused by an underlying hormonal condition. Stopping the use of medication or making use of alternative solutions can be risky.

All-around improvement in life

It is a fact that following this Adrenal Reset Power Boost Diet it is possible to notice and feel improvements in your daily life. You'll feel the improvements you've been waiting for to see happen:

1. You'll be more energetic throughout during the days when you require a boost. You'll be able to accomplish all sorts of things with the new energy and enthusiasm for the world around you.

2. You'll be able to be able to think clearly and take decisions. You will not have to worry about having a blurred mind that can affect your judgement at work or at schools.

3. You'll be able to recover from illness with ease, unlike before when a cold might bring you down. The stress and illnesses are normal circumstances in life, so you have to be resilient to bounce back unharmed. With this plan of diet it is possible to restore your the immune

system and health of your endocrine system.

4. You can enjoy prolonged periods awake, as well as a more peaceful sleep when you follow this Adrenal Reset Power Boost Diet program.

What foods to do and not consume

It is important to know you are following it is the Adrenal Reset Power Boost Diet is more than eating the right types of food and staying clear of the unhealthy ones. It's about eating the right foods at the right time and following a healthy schedule for eating every day. Here's a list with the best foods to choose from.

Food items you should be eating:

Super foods

1. Boost your immune system health.

2. Improve your digestion as well as your body's metabolism for food.

3. Enhance your energy levels to give you the energy you require throughout the day.

4. Enhance your appetite. Superfoods are tasty and delicious and are also extremely healthy.

5. Reduce your exposure to toxic substances when you eat foods that are organic, natural and not processed.

* Acai juice

* Apples

* Asparagus

* Avocado

* Blackberries

* Broccoli

* Brown rice

* Cauliflower

* Celtic sea salt

* Turkey and chicken

* Coconut

* Fatty fish like wild-caught salmon

* Seaweed and Kelp

* Kiwi

* Nuts, like almonds and walnuts

* Olives

* Oysters

* Peanut butter

* Sardines

* Scallops

* Seeds, including pumpkin and chia

* Soy milk

* Oats cut with steel

* Strawberries

* Sweet potatoes

High calorie foods

Oils, fats beef tallow, lard and fish oil:

Serving size: 902 calories/ 100 grams

(per cup: 1849 calories / 205 grams)

(per tablespoon: 117 calories / 13 grams)

Alternatives alternatives include: Soybean oil and coconut oil, walnut oil

Nuts, seeds, Macadamia nuts:

Serving size: 718 calories per 100 grams

(per cup: 948 calories/132 grams)

(per tablespoon: 201 calories/ 28 grams)

Alternatives: Pecans cashew nuts, pine nuts, flaxseeds and chia seeds

Dark Chocolate (70-85% cacao):

Serving size serving size: 598 calories/100 grams

(per cup: 604 calories/ 101 grams)

(per tablespoon: 167 calories/ 28 grams)

Alternative options Dark chocolate made of 60-69% cacao, and dark chocolate made with 45-59 percent cacao

Dried Fruit and juices of fruit (e.g. dried prunes/ prune juice):

Serving portion: 339 calories per 100 grams

(Per cup: 447 calories/ 132 grams)

(Per tablespoon (Per tablespoon): 224 calories/66 grams)

Alternative options: Dried blueberries, dried cherries, dried grape juice, dried peaches dried the juice of pomegranate and pineapple,

Avocados:

Serving size serving size: 160 calories/ 100 grams

(Per cup: 240 calories/ 150 grams)

(Per tablespoon (Per tablespoon: 332 calories/201 grams)

Whole grains, whole-wheat pasta cooked:

Serving Size: 124 calories/100 grams

(Per cup: 174 calories/ 140 grams)

(Per tablespoon (Per tablespoon): 87 calories/70 grams

Alternatives: Teff amaranth and spelt, quinoa Soba noodles, wild rice millet and bulgur.

Eggs, milk, and dairy goat's cheese hard:

Serving size Serving size: 452 calories/ 56 grams

(Per cup: 254 calories/ 56 grams)

(Per tablespoon (Per tablespoon: 127 calories/28 grams)

Alternative options Soft goat's cheese whole milk, feta, buttermilk Greek Yoghurt, protein powder, and Whey

oily fish, Mackerel, cooked:

Serving Size Serving Size: 262 calories/100 grams

(Per cup: 231 calories/ 88 grams)

(Per tablespoon): 223 calories(Per tablespoon: 223 calories / 85 grams

Alternative options: American shad, herring as well as trout, halibut tuna steak as well as tuna in canned oil, canned sardines and tuna steaks

Meat, Beef Brisket, cooked:

Serving portion Serving size: 358 calories/100 grams

(Per cup: 1124 calories/ 314 grams

(Per tablespoon (Per tablespoon: 304 calories/ 85 grams)

Alternative options Options include: Ground pork turkey bacon, turkey skin and meat and skin, veal loins as well as dark meat from chicken. drumsticks of chicken

Nutrient-dense foods

Vitamin B - rich foods

Foods high of vitamins B complex, particularly Vitamin B5 (or pantothenic acid) can improve the performance that the adrenal glands perform. Pantothenic acid deficiency could cause the adrenal glands to shrink and can result in them performing poorly, particularly during periods of stress.

The most potent sources for pantothenic acid include:

* Animal kidneys and the liver

* Avocados

* Broccoli

* Chicken

* Egg yolk

* Fish

* Legumes

* Milk

* Mushrooms

* Pork

* Shellfish

* Sweet potatoes

* Yogurt

Vitamin C - rich foods

Vitamin C is essential for the body to increase immunity, enhance the health of your cardiovascular system and improve the health of the adrenal glands. Vitamin C is required from the adrenal glands to make cortisol, which is needed during times of stress.

The following are fantastic Vitamin C sources:

* Berries

* Broccoli

* Brussels sprouts

* Mangoes

* Peaches

* Spring greens

* Tomatoes

L-tyrosine - rich foods

L-tyrosine helps to lessen the effect of stress on glands. It is crucial to ease the stress over the glands of adrenaline, so that they recover and be healthier.

These foods are high in L-tyrosine

* Avocados

* Bananas

* Chicken

* Dairy products

* Fish

* Legumes

* Nuts

* Oats

* Pork

* Seeds

* Wheat

* Whole grains

Supplements with nutritional value are another method of obtaining these nutrients. For those who don't are able to access the highest quality and most nutritious food choices can boost their intake of nutrients through the help of supplements. Ask your doctor to get advice on the most effective supplement brands that are suitable for you.

Probiotics

Lactobacillus is a popular probiotic that is present in yogurt as well as in fermented food items. This kind of probiotic could assist people who are prone to diarrhea or who are unable to handle lactose found in milk.

Bifidobacterium is a probiotic present in a variety of dairy products. It is helpful for those suffering from IBS, also known as irritable bowel syndrome (IBS).

The Role of Water

The body is cleansed with water, both in and out. It is the most essential element of the human body and is present in cells of the body as well as mucous membranes. The human body is comprised of around

3/4 water, therefore it is sensible that we drink the most water as feasible every day.

It is also possible to drink organic fruit juices as well as soups and gelatins and eat fruit that is that are high in water. It is vital to drink enough water as dehydration can strain the body. Being hydrated throughout the day boosts the adrenals' capacity to heal and recover from stress.

Food You Should Avoid

There are some food items you must avoid when on your Adrenal Reset Power Boost Diet.

Certain foods that you might be sensitive to

1. What is the primary ingredient? Do you think it contains any ingredients or food item that you are allergic to?

2. If you know the kind of food you getting, but remain concerned about the possibility of allergies, avoid the food, or consume just a little.

3. Look out for signs after you've had some bites.

4. Make sure you choose fresh, natural and free of toxins. Certain sufferers are more sensitive to certain foods than others. For some, even the tiniest quantities of chemicals and toxic substances can trigger an allergies. It's safer to be cautious than to risk being sorry.

5. Consult your physician about your allergies and ways to manage the symptoms. The more you're aware of the triggers of your allergy the better capable of avoiding straining the adrenal glands.

Caffeine

Sugar and sweeteners

Processed, artificially-prepared food items

Almost all processed and artificially-prepared foods are loaded with preservatives and chemicals that will not just tax the adrenals, but may make your symptoms worse. Make an effort to cook and prepare your own food. Avoid dining out and ordering take-away. If you shop, cook and cooking your own meals at home you will be able to significantly cut down on the consumption of processed food and, as an added bonus! - improve your cooking skills.

Chapter 10: How To Prevent Occupational Burnout In The Future

The saying goes: alter the circumstances. If you're unable to make a difference, you must modify yourself.

In this case also. If you're able to, you should change what's bothering your. It could be related to your work, colleagues and your position in the workplace. If you're unable to exert control over them or you don't want to alter them, you must modify something in you, your perspective, beliefs and focus, your attitude or your mental state. Whatever the situation, don't let the same circumstances cause you to be exhausted again.

Everything we've covered in this article will help you get over stress and help you regain your equilibrium. However, you must incorporate these ideas into your daily routine to ensure that it doesn't happen over and over. Also, you must be able to live a balanced and healthy lifestyle that is active in all aspects making sure that your goals are in line with your beliefs. If you have a solid base, there is no way to result in burnout and you'll never allow your work to be the sole thing you want to do.

In short, you have to look after your entire life and not just as a time to do work. Make sure you take the care of your body your mind, and your spirit Build relationships, nourish your soul, and earn for a living. Not just the opposite.

When you're aware of the significance of everything that's on your list of priorities, you'll are aware of what is most important over something other than that, and it's simple to determine where you should focus your attention and resources. Work shouldn't just be all that counts for you. It shouldn't cost your health, relationships or your happiness.

When you see a vision of your ideal life you've got a north star. You can stop anytime and ask yourself, does this lead me to my dream or draw me further from it? That way, you'll know what you need to do. If the longer hours at work actually make you feel closer to your goal, you'll be able take on them without feeling exhausted. If they result in losing your health, or a day of the school event of your child, that's far from your ideal life.

It is the temple of your body. Give it respect and appreciation. Nobody who is devoted to their body will be forced to be glued to the computer for hours. Do not degrade your body or nourish it with junk food or make it starve. Do not force your body to remain alert in the name of work. Don't let stress overwhelm you.

Slow down. Breathe. Be aware. Take as much rest as you're able to. Keep your body nourished with healthy foods. Drink plenty of water. Your brain is composed from a large amount of water. If you're hydrated your mind is clear. Move your body, stretch it out, exercise frequently, walk. There's no cost to exertion. Nobody will be rewarded for pushing yourself to the limit and making your body suffer--for what? Make sure you take care of your body and the one you've got.

Mental hygiene is essential and everyone must do it in order to be content. Being aware of your emotions and thoughts can be the very first thing you do toward harmony and peace within yourself. Every change you'd like to see in your physical world start within your head. It is therefore crucial to examine your beliefs, discover how to control your thoughts and control your emotions. In this way, you can become the master of your thoughts and your life instead of bouncing around on autopilot.

There are many methods to improve your mental health. Start by reading books about the topic, or even videos or podcasts, yoga meditation, self-development techniques, and tools.

If you are too focused on work, it may feel like the spin of a hamster's wheel, or participating in a race. Pause the computer. Take off the steering wheel. Relax, take a deep breath and then relax. It's not necessary to be constantly stressed. You don't need to be working all day long. You don't need to hurry.

Pause for a moment. Relax and recharge. After that, reorganize your schedule. Consider what you really want and what your soul desires. In the silence by the sea, in nature, or in contemplation. All of us need time to process our thoughts and feelings, but often we lack it due to the fact that we don't have the time. Allow yourself to spend as much time as you want, look at things as they are and be truthful about yourself.

Get rid of the "musts" and "have tos." The world will never cease to spin. There's nothing that can be done to stop it. Be patient, take in the environment around you as well as inside you and take note of it. If you are feeling refreshed and renewed, you can regain your control, put your life into your own hands and make a decision on everything that goes into it. This includes your job and priorities along with your dreams, both big and small goals, and each moment of your life. Be aware of your feelings and let your heart guide you to places and things that feel like home.

Chapter 11: Dealing With Different Stress Conditions

One of the results when you are subjected to stressful situations is an rise in cortisol levels. Cortisol levels that are elevated can lead to many issues.

Effect of Increased Cortisol Levels

Brain Function Gets Damaged

This is because cortisol interacts the memory directly. If this occurs the brain is afflicted with fog. which is a form of mental fog.

Cushing's Syndrome

There are a few rare cases of Cushing's syndrome patients. It's a serious but uncommon disease.

Weight Gain

As cortisol levels rise it boosts the appetite of the person. Additionally, cortisol signalizes your body that it is storing fats and thus the metabolic processes shift towards that direction.

Experience Tiredness

Cortisol is a factor that can disrupt the cycle of all hormones. This can cause disturbances in sleep and leave people tired.

Chronic Problems

There are many possible complications such as Type 2 osteoporosis, diabetes, and hypertension.

Because of its effect in the body's immune system the patient is more susceptible to getting sick.

It isn't necessary to be confused by all this. It is possible to take steps to decrease cortisol levels. Here are some tips for relaxation, diet and lifestyle suggestions which will assist you in reducing the amount of cortisol that is present in your body.

Corrective Action for High Cortisol Levels

Be cautious about Stressful Thinking

Cortisol release starts with stress-related thinking. It is essential to identify this warning sign and take appropriate actions. The group consisted of 122 participants, and instructed them to write about their previous negative events. The levels of cortisol increased over the course of a month opposed to those who wrote about things that were positive or created pleasant daily plans (Roos, Levens, & Bennett (2018)).

Being mindful and reducing stress is a good way to handle this problem. First step to be more aware of thoughts that trigger stress. Replace them with thoughts that are focused on positive things. Begin by acknowledging the thoughts that cause stress and negative feelings.

Undergo Training in Self-Awareness

Train yourself to become conscious of your thoughts and breathing, beginning by listening to your heartbeat. You will then become aware of stress and the moment at which it starts. The awareness allows you to become an observer of your emotions , instead of being a passive victim.

If one is aware of worrying thoughts, it is possible to create a strategy to combat them by planning deliberate responses to each thought that is stressful. A group of women who underwent mindfulness classes showed that an individual's ability to accurately describe stress was directly associated with lower levels of cortisol. A different group of over 100 breast cancer patients found that mindfulness training can reduce cortisol levels, when compared to a the absence of a stress management program.

In short, mindfulness of stress aids in self-awareness and helps individuals to identify symptoms and reduce tension in the body. It is essential to start by being aware of the triggers that stress can cause and this can help you deal effectively with stress.

Be Sure to Get Enough Sleep

Cortisol is heavily influenced by the length, timing in addition to the level of quality sleep. In observing a set working shifts, the researchers observed that cortisol levels were greater when people slept throughout the daytime. In addition, sleep deprivation resulted in elevated levels of cortisol over a prolonged period.

The regular daily pattern of hormone levels were disrupted due to shift rotations. This caused fatigue to increase and various other issues because of high cortisol levels. The insomnia condition due to high cortisol levels can last for up to 24 hours at minimum. A brief interruption in sleep could raise levels and disrupt the pattern of hormones that we experience daily. If you are working an hourly shift that rotates or your night shift you won't be able to control your sleeping. You can improve the quality of your rest by following a few steps.

A) Avoid drinking caffeine in the evening If you consume tea or coffee during the evening or late at night, it could cause you to be awake.

B) Do not do any thrilling activities prior to bed. By staying clear of distractions before your bedtime, you will be able to ensure your mind is at peace. A peaceful mind can enhance the quality of your sleep. Utilize earplugs to block out white noise , and avoid taking liquids prior to sleep.

c) Do not use bright lights limit exposure to bright lights by using shades and screens. A dark space helps your mind relax and provides you with a restful sleep.

d) Perform some exercises Keep active physically throughout the daytime. This will aid in getting better sleep.

e) Take napping: If you work shifts, then naps could help reduce the amount of sleep you need. Utilize short naps when you can.

In short, a regular sleeping schedule can help you stay clear of distractions and interruptions to your sleep and ensure you get at least 8 to 7-8 hours of rest each day. This can help keep cortisol levels at a healthy level.

Get a Pet

Interacting with your pet can reduce cortisol levels. The researchers observed that stress-related conditions improved when one employed therapy dogs. Additionally, therapy dogs kept cortisol levels in check in children who underwent medical procedures.

They also observed that spending time with dogs offered more emotional support than interacting with a person. When interacting of the animal, the individual could ease the tensions of the social environment and be more peaceful. In another instance they studied the effect of cortisol in reducing stress having the dog. They compared it to an uncontrolled group that didn't have pets. The pet owners did not show significant reductions in cortisol levels after they had dogs. As pet owners have already enjoyed this benefit, they didn't exhibit any significant differences during the research.

Aside from that The animals also enjoyed the advantages from positive interaction. It was evident that the bond between animals was beneficial to both.

In short, interaction with animals can reduce stress. This can result in less cortisol levels. Pets also enjoy interacting with humans.

Wow! Congratulations!

Chapter 12: Stress Management Techniques

We've all been through difficult times in our lives. Some were simple to manage and others more challenging. We all react and feel differently when faced with stressful situations. So, there are not all strategies to manage stress that are equally effective for everyone. What is stressful for you doesn't have to be stressful for who is not. Therefore, we'll show the most popular ones because they have as per some studies proven to be the most effective. The most important thing is it for you to discover and apply the ones that are most suitable for you.

We'll begin with a few types that of stress-management macro methods and will then go over more specific steps. The first step to manage stress, like in dealing with any other issue is to identify the causes of stress. It is then about finding ways to remove these triggers, and lessen the amount of stress and the final step is to understand how to reduce and prevent stress in the future.

How do we identify the source of stress? How can you get rid of it and keep from stress-inducing situations in the future?

Sometimes, it's pretty obvious which direction your stress is coming from. When you are in certain situations such as being married, having child or facing the death of a loved ones, you're even putting your trust in stress, and you are preparing yourself to combat and ease the stress. However, there are instances where it's just not obvious what the root of your stress. In this scenario, you'll be able to trace your stress to the root of it.

To be more precise in the case of stressors, we'll categorize them as internal and external stressors.

External stressors are the instances or events that originate from your environment that impact your mood, attitude and behavior. There are a myriad of external stressors that we experience every day. For instance, big life transitions could be the cause of anxiety - such as a new marriage, a planned baby, new home and so on. If these changes require more work, when they are burdensome and we are unable to cope the stress, it could lead to an emotional breakdown. Certain inputs from our surroundings including the sudden sound of traffic or even the barking dogs, are thought to be external stressors. Work stress, pressing deadlines, a boss who is demanding and other unpredictable circumstances can all cause stress. Being around new people and feeling uncomfortable due to that or, for example going out on a blind date can be for many people extremely stressful circumstances.

Stressors that are internal, like their name implies, come from within, and are emotionally or psychological triggers of stress. Internal stressors are thoughts and emotions that come up in our minds in response to a particular reason and cause us to feel anxious and restless. It is interesting to note that internal stress doesn't originate with an an external stressors even though we could think of some. It is a result of a myriad of anxiety (fear that of speaking in public, fear failing or flying etc.).

You can, for instance, take a notebook and note down all the factors that cause you feel stressed, the triggers, or stressors. Once you've compiled a list of the stressful events and you've written them down, you can record the way you responded and the actions you took to ease the anxiety. It is also possible to write down the likely stressors that you're going to have to confront and then begin to think of strategies to minimize the stress. The process of identifying your stress allows you to determine the amount of anxiety you felt in specific circumstances.

In recognizing a problem and in identifying the root of stress, you've made the first step towards improving your ability to manage stress in the future. Now is the time to take the next step.

The second part is to explore the various options you have to manage stress. There are a lot of options and we're certain you'll find the ones which work for you. In order to find the most effective strategies to deal with stress, we'll discuss the specific scenarios that are thought stress-inducing. They include stressed at work, anxiety at college and relationships, stress, the stress of being in a relationship, and stress from environmental sources. If you find yourself in any of these stressful situations, it is possible to explore your options and try some of the strategies we have provided. These tips will assist you in dealing with stress when it's present.

The third step to a stress-free and peaceful life is obviously, learning how to reduce stress and anxiety and eliminate anxiety from your life. It's not an easy task because it requires time. In order to get as close as you can to a stress-free living, the main focus should be focused on yourself. That means you have be thinking about yourself first. This may sound selfish, however it's not. If you can manage stress, when you can maintain your calm and calm and perform better, and will positively impact your surroundings. Being in well-balanced physical and mental condition is vital not just for productivity, but also for the overall atmosphere of your home or workplace as your attitude greatly influences the those in your vicinity. Consider this: There are people in your life that tend to be negative and pessimistic. What do they affect you? How does their behavior influence your mood? Sure! Be sure not to be one of them. Be positive and learn to manage anxiety will make you stronger and make you better able to assist and inspire others around you.

Chapter 13: Sleep To Be Young: How Sleep Helps Slow Aging?

It's not a secret that getting enough rest is beneficial for your well-being. Research has revealed that sleeping can slow the aging process and make you look younger for a longer duration.

Melatonin the sleep hormone is what helps us to sleep through the night. It plays a role in regulating our body's clock, as well as other essential functions. Through lengthy study it has been found to be beneficial in combating heart disease and diabetes. It also aids in promoting bone health and reduces the risk of weight gain. Recent research has also revealed that this hormone is able to protect your body's DNA as well as help prevent the decline of aging and diseases.

Melatonin is produced by the pineal gland. It has a transducing capacity, and it releases into the bloodstream in the dark and can help induce sleep. The body naturally produces more of melatonin and this is why they are more likely to fall asleep. As we age, production of melatonin declines and it becomes harder to sleep.

As you age one night of poor sleep can be seen in your face. The skin may lose its shape, develop bags, or appear dull. Sleeping in can make you appear ten years older. The facial tissues need relaxation from stress in order to renew. Beauty sleep isn't just a cliche.

While you sleep, growth hormones help stimulate the repair of cells and tissues. Lack of sleep can impede regeneration and result in the accelerated aging process. It also increases cortisol levels and cause worsening of inflammation-related disorders. If you are feeling restless in the time of night, your body might be swelling because of the extra fluid. The recommended amount of time can help your body to eliminate the excess fluid, while also repairing the skin. Collagen does not form correctly in the same way.

Collagen aids in giving the skin its shape, gets rid of dead cells and encourages the growth of new cells on the skin. The protein is created when you rest. It prevents the development of wrinkles. It also increases the flexibility of the skin. A good night's sleep can reduce inflammation and swelling.

Sleep deprivation also causes more oxidative stress, which could lead to premature ageing and poor skin. A buildup of lymphatic fluid and inadequate drainage can also cause puffy eyes or dark circles.

Chapter 14: Why You Need A Meaning To Your Life

"The mystery of human existence lies not in just staying alive, but in finding something to live for." The author is Fyodor Dostoyevsky

There have been numerous studies that have examined the negative effects of stress, and the results of these studies are that without doubt, if there is a some meaning in your life and understand the significance of your life You will be less likely be afflicted by stress. Also, you're more likely to be able to stay longer in your life and be healthier. It is possible to look at various lifestyles and it's logical that people with satisfaction with the purpose for their existence are much less likely be suffering from health problems such as:

There are people who are able to fight off the flu each winter. It's not an accident.

They take care of themselves and are self-careful because they are driven in life and are aware that they must fulfill the goal. Therefore, they are less likely to take advantage of either their minds or bodies, and are more responsible to the wellbeing and health of their family members. The same is true for older people living with a partner because their lives are more rational while someone who lives on their own and without visitors might think that their lives have limited value. Being alone as you get old is a scary experience and can result in stress as it is the time of year when illnesses are likely become more probable.

For the pensioner who is old or senior citizen living alone pet ownership has been proven beneficial for a variety of reasons. It provides them with the motivation to rise each day and gives them an element of accountability towards someone else than themselves. Pets require food and so the senior is likely to be more likely to follow the same routine. The fact that there is something to look after aside from oneself can be a huge help in such situations as it provides the senior with life a meaning they might not have the ability to access.

In reality, if you look at those who retired early usually, they die prematurely because they've lost the significance of their lives, and there is no reason to live for them anymore. But it doesn't have to be this way. If you're planning to retire such a scenario it could give enough reasons to be excited about it. However, many people don't think that in the same way, particularly when premature retirement can make them feel inadequate. A forced early retirement because of medical issues could have the same negative consequences. Therefore, it can be seen from this that finding meaning to your life is essential even if it is just getting together with your friends at the golf course or tending to the garden.

People looking for an explanation for their lives could be at any age any time. Teenagers may be affected by the loss of a loved one and it brings home how small life can be and make life appear unimportant for them. Couples who have broken up and they are left there is no normal family routine They feel that the purpose of their lives have been taken away from their feet, which can lead to extreme anxiety. Children can also feel that the world is meaningless when confronted with situations which are challenging for them. They may be unable to pass their school exams or show signs of signs of a decrease in their abilities to learn that could be attributed to stress.

People who aren't connected to their lives can easily slip into the anxiety that comes with the seemingly meaningless life they lead. People who are in dire situations might have needs in their lives, but they don't necessarily believe that their lives are insignificant. When you examine some examples of the behaviors of those who have suffered from tragedy, for example you might be wondering what they will be living for. These people will amaze you due to the fact that their purpose in life is heightened because of their tragic experiences. They are elated to be alive and will strive to restore the structure of their lives. This is due to their desire to live on. The people who are in situations like they are extremely strong and may not have time to be stressed. They are too busy reestablishing their lives.

A few people locate their purpose in the people who surround them, but it's not wise to rely on that all the time. In the event that the loved ones die and they are unable to fulfill their purpose and, as a result, are in a position of not having an excuse to continue. They are the ones who have to discover their purpose, because until they do they'll have a difficult time being content and get rid of the cycle of negative thoughts that causes stress.

This is why it's essential to know your identity and what you're capable of and aim towards goals and goals. It is essential to establish an area of focus in your life since when you have one, it's easier to get rid from stress. It's as if it provides you with an initial point of reference. Once you've found that starting point and you have that, you'll also have the motivation to be positive and work towards an optimistic future and allows little space for anxiety to play a role in it. People who are entrepreneurs or have discovered their motivation in life will realize that they thrive when challenged and have a reason for their lives, and the meaning they give to their lives is the reason they are able to keep going and how they stay optimistic in their outlook.

Find your goal and practice it.

If you think that life is a waste of time it is time to give your life a some sense of. Everyone has a reason to live our lives and it is your responsibility to figure out what it is that you are looking for and work on them until they actually provide you with a reason to put aside your worries and begin having fun. There's a lot of happiness waiting to be experienced by you it. At present take note of what you believe the meaning of your life. What are the things you accomplish or contribute to the world? It may appear dull at first, but it is important to enhance it with the beauty that these activities contribute to your daily life. For instance:

I'm passionate about what I do I take lots of enjoyment from my work.

I love my children. My children are my most enjoyable thing in my life.

I love getting up and take care of my canaries. They're stunning, exquisite and beautiful creatures.

It is possible that you are not taking advantage of things you are blessed with that others don't. If you think about your lifestyle with a lot of detail, then you will decide which activities bring satisfaction to you. These are the things that bring joy to your experience. What are the things that make you unhappy? These are things that drain your purpose and meaning. If there's a way for you to avoid doing things that bring you no joy and replace them with positive activities and actions, this will allow you see the purpose behind your actions.

Remember that the goal of your existence isn't dependent on what you have. They are things that will pass away and your life is not defined by the things you own. It is important to figure out what motivates you to get up each morning and, if you see no purpose in your life Try to find new reasons to rise. Set yourself goals to complete. Set small goals, even though they aren't your primary goal but they can contribute to it and can help you gain the confidence to find what you are looking for in life.

Chapter 15: Underlying Causes

There are many underlying problems that could cause constant and constant discomfort. These include nutrition, metabolism as well as infections and toxic issues.

Nutrition - Low in ferritin, B12, Folic acid, hydroxy Vitamin B1, D1, and C

Metabolism - Adrenal Dysfunction and Hyperthyroidism

Infections It can be caused by Hepatitis C, Lyme disease or co-infections with parasites, an overgrowth of bacteria in the gut and enteroviruses

Toxic issues related to jet fuel, heavy metals , pesticides

Stress and Hormones

Hormones are vital to living a healthy life. The master gland, also known as the hypothalamus is the one responsible for sending biochemical signals to our thyroid gland and pituitary gland, adrenal glands and even the Ovaries. The hypothalamus regulates the metabolism rate, the immune system and the nervous system autonomic and many other things. The body's tissues send chemical messages back to the gland that controls them. The information loops and messages impact the symptoms seen in Fibromyalgia.

There is evidence of the hormonal sequence is disrupted in patients suffering from Fibromyalgia. A problem in one region can affect other areas. Experts have discovered such disturbances in environmental and genetic influences, as and psychological stress.

Thyroid Gland Thyroid Gland tension in thyroid hormones, this may be due to unbalanced adrenal gland. Studies have proven the connection with Fibromyalgia and thyroid disorders that are particularly prevalent in women who are menopausal. Signs of a weak immunity as well as low body temperature and fatigue may contribute to the severity of Fibromyalgia. Treatment for hyperthyroidism can help alleviate the symptoms of Fibro.

Adrenal glands that release cortisol is their main purpose. There is a cycle in our daily lives of cortisol, which we release when in stress. People with Fibromyalgia typically report feeling overwhelmed by stress, more likely due to the imbalance. There have been studies that suggest there's a link between cortisol rhythms that are disrupted and emotional trauma in those suffering from Fibromyalgia. The support of one's adrenal health and healing toxic emotions can boost your stress-response of the person. Furthermore, it will enhance the ability to deal with the symptoms of fibro.

Ovaries - women who suffer from fibro generally suffer from more severe symptoms both during menstrual cycles and post-menstrual. This is due to hormones testosterone, estrogen and progesterone, which impact the body's symptoms of fatigue and pain. If you can regulate your hormones through thyroid, adrenal and ovarian stimulation, it will help to lessen the symptoms of fibro, and the condition is likely to improve while also reducing symptoms and learning strategies to cope.

Central Sensitization Theory

Fibro patients tend to experience more severe discomfort. While the reason behind this is still unknown however, there are a variety of studies that could explain the reason. Researchers and scientists have concluded that the pain originates in the tissues deep beneath the joints and muscles. Sleep deprivation is the result of tightening muscles. In the absence of adequate rest, muscles won't be able recover. This could result in the continual signals being sent to the central nervous system as well as muscles. This affects how your central nervous system interprets external factors. The patient is then more sensitive and prone to pain, also known as central sensitization.

What's fascinating about these events is that the symptoms and causes of Fibromyalgia are thought as bidirectional. The imbalances could cause muscles to contract, which may also cause structural imbalances. Also, sleep deprivation could cause tightening of muscles and the tightening of muscles can result in sleep problems. This is it's a vicious cycle. A person can prevent this by making sure that she's getting the proper nutrition and appropriate amount of rest that helps maintain the muscle's performance optimally.

Chapter 16: My Happy Body
SMOOTHIES AND SUPER-GREEN DRINKS

Smoothies made from fruits and vegetables can be a simple method to provide your body with vital nutrients. The best method to determine the precise ingredients of your smoothie is to prepare the smoothie yourself. All you require is blenders, fruits vegetables, as well as the base of your choice, like yogurt, milk, or water. The process of making your own juices could aid in preventing fruits and vegetables from being wasted and also provide advantages that help you stay on the path to better health.

Each of the options above will provide you with the daily requirements of nutrients and vitamins that your body requires to flourish. In just 15 minutes after drinking a raw juice of a vegetable, we absorb and digest the nutrients that provide nourishment and regenerative power to tissues, glands, cells and organs within our body. When we consume cooked vegetables or steam-cooked with other foods it could take anywhere from 3-4 days to digest, and absorb.

Blending smoothies with frozen organic fruits, a handful of veggies from your fridge and a small amount of organic yogurt is a great method to replenish your nutrition between meals. The antioxidants in berries reduce inflammation. Include a few citrus fruits because they're loaded with Vitamin C.

Mix celery, parsley, and spinach to make a smoothie or juice and add a bit of ginger with lemon and you'll be energized for many hours. You could lose some pounds easily because you'll not feel the urge to overeat during mealtimes.

Take care not to drink too much smoothies that are fruit-based due to the sugar content.

Always add natural yogurt that balances the digestive system.

Let's celebrate your body's happiness!

ZEAL - ALL IN ONE

Many years ago, I was told by a Naturopath that there wasn't enough vitamins, minerals , and antioxidants contained in Protein powders we consume. He even said those like me who mixed smoothies had to add fish-oils to heart health, and milk thistle to support liver health, and a small amount of kelp to shield us from exposure to radiation. Gingko for memory, plus B vitamin for the nervous system , an extra Cwith Niacin to boost the immune system and of course Efor the skin, and D-3 with calcium to strengthen bones. The reason behind all of the additional supplements was that in more than 25 years of the practice, every person who visited my doctor's clinic was nutritionally deficient, and he was extremely worried about our health.

To put it mildly it's been a hassle through the years. Most times I've utilized the supplements of herbs and vitamins the doctor suggested to put in my smoothies or protein drinks. It's a time-consuming process and costs money around $250.00 monthly, but it is effective.

It's true that in the long run it's cheaper to remain healthy than to get sick. We've all heard of people who have a serious disease, and the price for insurance coverage is astronomical.

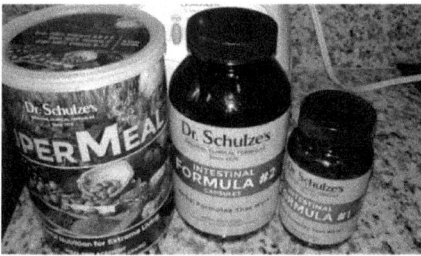

I recently was introduced to the Wellness formula ZAL- which was claimed to have minerals, vitamins and antioxidants, as well as herbs as well as enzymes and prebiotics. I was a bit skeptical as I wasn't sure it had sufficient of the ingredients to have a significant impact. So I retreated to the cold and stopped taking all of my supplements in order to give ZEAL an opportunity and give it to give it a run for its money.

I'm here to tell you that it is working. I started with one breakfast serving. I then had an additional serving in the afternoon. My energy level increased. I'm focused throughout the day and am more stamina-ful than I have ever had before. After the third day of taking two servings I had to reduce down to one serving, that is 1 scoop in 8 ounces of water. I've been using 1 scoop daily, but without adding the additional supplements as they're included in ZEAL. I'm saving time and money. one month's supply costs $59.95 as the preferred customer. I could not join up quickly enough.

I make smoothies on weekend, but I do not need to add individual vitamins and herbs to it. I take Zeal every morning before breakfast and then keep the portions in my car for when I require a an energy boost in later afternoon.

I am thankful of my buddy Dave who introduced my family and me to Zeal because it's the genuine. I fully endorse the product and would like you to try it. www.ellacroney.zealforlife.com

Contact me for any questions:

CLEAN THE INSIDE OUT

MILK THISTLE: This herb is often utilized as a natural remedy for liver issues. The causes of liver problems are jaundice, cirrhosis, hepatitis and gallbladder problems.

Certain claims Milk Thistle may also:

It cleanses and protects your liver. It is also known to be the "liver rejuvenator. The liver is an important blood reservoir, that removes toxins from us each and every minute. If you are feeling exhausted after eating, or after drinking a sweet coffee drink or soda, and you often feel angry or angry with no cause in particular, your liver may be under stress. Utilizing this herb, Milk Thistle can do wonders for you.

Find it at Trader Joes or a high quality Health food store to be sure there aren't any additives added. Always check with your doctor to determine whether Milk Thistle may be beneficial for you.

INTESTINAL FORMULA #1

The fantastic advantages from this supplement I wrote about the amazing benefits of this product in (FOREVER Young) and I wanted to give it to you because it is so effective. This herb-based product as well as numerous others is an invention by Dr. Schulze's herbal pharmacy.

I have used his products throughout my time as I was a flight attendant. They aid in the elimination of high levels of radiation and heavy metals out my body. These products are more powerful than the words. Patients have been cured of serious illnesses, and some had been on their deathbeds when a loving family member or friend initiated them on The Dr. Schulze's remedies.

Everyone begins at Intestinal Formula #1 - because it helps to maintain regular and full stool movements. This product increases and strengthens the muscle movement of the colon. It helps cleanse and rid your body of the accumulated waste. I can assure you that it does the trick!

Based on the research of the doctor Dr. Schulze, "the average American has between 10 and 12 pounds of fecal matter the colon. If this waste isn't cleared out regularly, it could make your body filled with poisons, which can make it slow as well as unhealthy."

What you take out of your home is just as important as the things you do with it. Enjoy your cleansing!

Chapter 17: Other Effective Tips

In addition to the suggestions mentioned in the previous chapters you could also try some of these helpful techniques that will help you increase your energy levels and combat fatigue. Take a look at the other paragraphs below.

Release negative feelings

Anger and sadness take away your energy, and it is best to get rid of them as soon as you can. The best thing will help you is identify the root of these emotions and then deal effectively. If you are suffering from issues with your anger management and depression issues, then you might require the assistance from an expert. This is, naturally difficult to do however it is crucial to take action on your negative feelings to prevent your mind from being exhausted. In addition to sadness and anger other emotions that sap out energy are frustration and jealousy, envy sadness, anger as well as despair, doubt and doubt. Learn to feel and think positively to boost your energy levels and combat fatigue.

Have more sexual sex

Engaging in regular sexual activity can improve your energy levels as well as combat fatigue. When you're engaging in sexual activity in a relationship with someone else, the entire body is activated. Sexual activity burns calories, increases immunity, and increases oxygenation. It's also a fantastic relaxation tool and helps reduce anxiety. Sexual stimulation can be a great source of energy this is the reason why experts suggest couples perform it at the beginning of the day to keep them energized through the entire day. If you believe that you don't have the passion you experienced in your younger years, take into consideration getting your testosterone levels tested since this hormone is responsible for sex drive for both genders. It increases libido and boosts the level of energy.

Get ready for your menstrual cycle for women

Women experience an imbalance of hormones at least once a month during PMS. They go into a rage during this particular period during the month. This hormonal imbalance may create fatigue. Women must prepare themselves for this by eating lots of complex carbohydrates and fiber in the form of vegetables, fruits as well as whole grain. Also, they should avoid salt and caffeine, and do more exercise. Men must also be prepared for the period of time if they live with a female. Living with a woman who is having a period is like living in the edge of a volcano, which is set to explode at any moment and this can be exhausting on its own.

Think about your age

It is likely that as you get older, you'll become less active. It will be harder to perform the things you did while in your

20s, now that you're older. It is important to take into consideration your age when exercising. For instance, if reach your 60th birthday and would like to climb mountains do not put too much pressure on yourself if you are tired easily. It is not a good idea to make yourself do things that are difficult for your body's natural capabilities.

Listen to the music

If you're feeling exhausted and sleepy , and aren't feeling motivated to do anything play some upbeat music that instantly boosts your energy. You can listen to hip hop and dance music that will inspire you to be more energetic. It is possible to do this in the morning when you're preparing to leave for work, or while cleaning the house. You can also enjoy beats when you exercise or run. However If you're looking to unwind and relax it is best to listen to relaxing music. This can be done after working for a long time or before the time you go to bed.

Consult a physician

If you've tried a variety of relaxation methods and lifestyle changes to reduce fatigue, but remain tired all the time It might be the right time to consult an expert. You may need to get your thyroid examined for issues that make you be tired constantly. You can have the blood test to get the total blood cell count to identify thyroid issues. You may also visit specialist to see for issues with vitamin or allergy which can explain why you are exhausted constantly.

Chapter 18: Available Treatment Programs

There are no cures for CFS however, there are many methods available to help sufferers overcome the signs of symptoms, signs and effects that have a significant impact not just on their physical appearance but also mental and emotional aspects as well. These treatments are based on the way in which the condition affects individuals.

A customized treatment plan must be available to every CFS patient in accordance with the National Institute for Health and Care Excellence. The program should be able to deal with physical and emotional effects of CFS to the patient , and ways to improve or maintain the patient's capabilities. Treatments can benefit one person, but not to the other , therefore all risk and benefit of every treatment should be discussed with the patient. The patient is entitled to decline the recommended treatment and seek alternative treatments that suits his/her needs.

Graded Exercise Therapy

A Graded Exercise Therapy or GET is an exercise regimen designed to gradually improve the patient's capacity to perform a specific physical exercise. It typically includes aerobic exercises and other activities that increase the heart rate, such as swimming and walking. The program of exercise is based on the individual's physical abilities.

It is best to be started by a qualified specialist and, as much as is possible it should be provided in a one-to-one manner. Once determining the baseline of a person or level of exercise gradually, the intensity of the exercise will rise.

A key part of the plan is setting goals with the therapy. It could be a few months, weeks, months, or even years for the patient to accomplish the goals , but it is essential that he stays to the given time and intensity and not go beyond the limit. In the beginning of the program, smaller tasks like gardening can be undertaken. The endurance and strength of the patient will increase over time.

Cognitive Behavioral Therapy

Cognitive Behavioral Therapy (CBT) is a different kind of therapy that assists in regulating the patient's behavior as well as their way of thinking. It is typically used for many ailments that seek to ease the intensity of symptoms. Furthermore, it's an important tool for breaking down the other overwhelming issues into smaller pieces by fighting the cycle of negative emotions thoughts, behaviors, and physical symptoms that are typical for patients with CFS.

The treatment plan is best delivered on a one-to one basis, and it is tailored to the needs of the patient. It could also include difficult thoughts that can aid the patient in preventing the symptoms from getting worse and assisting him to accept the diagnosis given and aiding in gaining control over his symptoms. The use of CBT to identify the chronic fatigue syndrome does not necessarily indicate that the patient is suffering from an emotional issue. It is often utilized to treat chronic illnesses like cancer and rheumatoid arthritis.

It is built on specialists' belief that the way people think thinking may lead to health issues. The therapy also aims to change harmful or ineffective behaviours. While it's not able to fix the disorder, it assists in improving its symptoms and searching for strategies that can be beneficial to the patient's everyday functioning. In general, CBT will include the creation of a goal, setting a schedules for sleep, managing daily activities, and providing psychological support.

Support System

Based on the severity of the condition depending on the severity of the condition, other forms of support could be required like nursing assistance medical equipment, caregivers and home modifications to deal with the disability of the patient. If you are employed, their doctor or health professional will guide them on when they should take time off from to rest and work. In addition, the patient may have to work a certain amount of hours , and also perform an additional assignment.

Additionally they are excellent sources of tips to help, advice and information for managing Chronic fatigue syndrome. You can also discuss your issues with others, ask questions, or express your feelings and frustrations throughout your treatment. Consult your physician about the closest group support you can get in touch with.

MANAGING RELAPSES

It is common to experience setsbacks or relapses, especially when the symptoms become more severe. They can be caused by numerous factors like an infection, sleep issues and stress. Discuss with your physician possible ways to treat and methods to use in the event of any relapses. Make sure to keep your workouts and activities to an absolute minimum. Practice relaxation techniques, and speak to your family and friends more frequently. In the event of a relapse, have to return to the previously-rested level of exercise.

When a patient is relapsing, their symptoms can become more severe, making the patient unable to perform the tasks he had previously manage. Many factors could trigger relapses, including extreme exercise and infections. The doctor can assist patients manage the relapses through regular breaks from their normal routine of exercise.

MANAGING ACTIVITIES

The ability to manage one's activities is another aspect that is covered in different treatment programs. It involves setting the patient's goals and gradually increasing the amount of physical activity. Keep a log of your daily activities and time between your rests to determine your base. Additionally, you should avoid vigorous activities or even increasing its intensity and duration over what you are able to manage.

Chapter 19: What Can I Eat To Boost My Testosterone Levels?

A hormone that has more effects than just your sexual drive, lower levels of testosterone should be given urgent attention, regardless of the age. Hypogonadism, which is a medical term used for low levels of testosterone, could be treated in a number of ways but whatever is the course of treatment, your doctor would suggest you to have a diet that is enriched with testosterone-boosting elements. Below are a few of foods you can try:

Vitamin D is known as a dazzling vitamin that functions quietly in many bodily functions, among that is the absorption of enough calcium to maintain strong bones and a healthy immune system. Vitamin D plays a crucial part in increasing testosterone levels. This is the reason why food that is enriched by Vitamin D is an effective method of increasing the testosterone. From eggs fortified with

Vitamin D and milk products, you are able to test the one that suits your taste.

A daily intake of tuna is a very efficient way to boost the T hormone. In addition, it is high of Vitamin D, adding to its efficacy. It is possible to choose canned or fresh tuna. A single serving of tuna per day is enough to cover equally your Vitamin D and testosterone levels.

Sardines and salmon are equally effective in boosting levels as tuna , however it is important to be aware that eating excessive levels of Omega-3 could result in prostate cancer in the future.

As mentioned earlier the proper amount of Vitamin D within the body will ensure that your T hormone remains stable. Shrimp could increase the Vitamin D levels, which increases the T hormone. This is another reason for you to head to the ocean to make the seafood you most beloved friend.

Pumpkin seeds are a great source of zinc that is directly connected to testosterone production within your body. People who have low zinc levels tend to have low levels of testosterone. Pumpkin seeds can be added to cereals, oatmeal as well as salads, and get your daily intake of vegetables. If you're not a fan to chew them up, consider adding them into smoothies for a nutritious diet.

Do you realize that the right fats can be a big help in helping to maintain high amounts of testosterone? Which better method to boost to them than by incorporating coconuts into your diet routine? Coconuts are a good source of balanced levels of saturated fat which can help keep your testosterone levels in check without overdoing it.

Minerals are important in the context of the hormone T and that's why magnesium plays a crucial role in regulating testosterone. Wheat bran is a fantastic source of magnesium, and can be a good source of T hormone when combined with regular workouts for strength.

Wheat bran is a great addition to shakes with protein or batter for pancakes, cookies or oatmeal porridge.

Ricotta cheese is a great source of protein from whey. When you work out hard, your body can inhibit the production of sexual hormones, and that's when the protein in whey comes in handy. It blocks the effects of the cortisol hormone released by your body in reaction to stress. It maintains the testosterone hormone in balance.

As well as being a powerful antioxidant, the strawberries are also loaded in Vitamin C that counters the effects of cortisol on the body. If you're stressed or overwhelmed by the demands of your job, your body could release cortisol which can further limit its capacity to produce testosterone. Incorporating strawberries into your diet can help aid in reducing cortisol.

It's not for naught that we have a name for honey "nature's healer". Boron which is an essential mineral in honey, is able to boost testosterone levels. Honey also has nitric oxide that can cause more powerful and lasting and more lasting erections.

Cabbage is a fantastic food. It's not just perfect for a quick vegetable stir-up, but it is also great for your testosterone-boosting strategies. Cabbage is rich in indole-3-carbinol, which reduce the effect of estrogen, a female hormone, in the body, thereby increasing the availability of testosterone and making it more efficient.

Staying engaged

It's definitely difficult to stay engaged in the numerous things you must do every day. If you're advised to take two pills a daily to do better at bedtime you are likely to some self-esteem issues that will keep you from doing what you should be doing. It's all about trusting in your body's capacity to overcome challenges and beat these. When you're making diet changes, don't think of it as something that is difficult rather, you should consider making the changes a part of your daily routine as a means towards a goal which will eventually lead to improved overall health.

There will be many reasons that pop up in your mind to not exercise today or eating that yummy pasta on the next day, but at conclusion of your day you'll need to be able to guide yourself to eating a healthy diet.

Chapter 20: Pearls

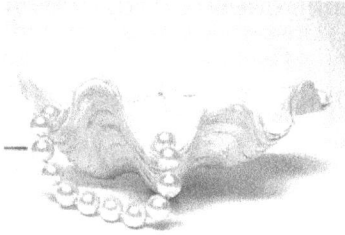

First Pearl -No ALA...

Do not take the supplement Alpha Lipoic Acid in the beginning of your detoxification. Examine your supplements, particularly the multivitamins and multiminerals. If the supplement has 10-20 mgs, it's not worth it. Follow this advice with a lot of care. In the past, I was taking 600 mgs of ALA when I was adhering to a doctor's plan. (I won't mention the name of the practitioner). I began to experience suicidal thoughts with severe insomnia and shaking. I stayed with this plan for a few days. I wasted my time and suffering. ALA is more than just an antioxidant, but it's a brain chelator to heavy metals, particularly mercury. Based on Andy Cutler, I was taking massive amounts of ALA which isn't recommended. I'm with him. ALA is able to penetrate the brain's blood barrier that can cause heavy metals, such as mercury to escape from the brain. If you're not in a proper chelation program the mercury will circulate back to the brain, which can cause a number of negative signs and symptoms, as was the case for me.

This is because the chemically sensitive people at the early stages of detoxification aren't ready to remove the metal from their brains.

Instead of beginning by cleansing your body and nutrition, ALA is now working to chelate your brain. Who would want to sprint straight to the brain's chelation?

Why do alternative doctors suggest ALA even though it's not an element of a chelation plan? Your answer is as reliable as mine. I promised you in my introduction that I would give you details. I delivered. Do not take ALA in any circumstance unless you are under the care of a doctor who is specialized in brain-chelation.

If a physician is performing IV chelation, leave the clinic. All chelators can be used either orally and in rectally. It's a risk to take IV Chelation.

Second Pearl - MarCons

It is a MarCons Nasal Swap test is essential for people who are sensitive to chemicals even if you don't suffer from sinus problems. Consult your physician "What is the MarCons test? She/he may be unsure. It is available on the internet costing $85.00. I took advantage of Microbiology DX to check the presence of MarCons. The price of that Nares Bacterial Culture comprises MarCons and other pathogens of bacterial origin is $85.00.

The request form stipulates that a doctor's recommendation is required, however you are able to stipulate on the form that the results will be delivered via your residence. If the request is not accepted, you can have your physician help you with the purchase. You could be teaching your child something brand new!

If you are unable to use an internet-connected device, the telephone number is 718-276-5057. They're found within Bedford, MA.

MarCons is "Multiple Antibiotic Resistant Coagulase Negative Staphylococcus." That's a mouthful! Before you take the test, check out the MarCons nasal swap test demonstration via You Tube. Boy! That's a good suggestion. You should follow the same process in case the nasal stick does not penetrate deep enough into the sinuses for an exact diagnosis. I did it, so be brave and do it too!

If you're MarCons tests are positive,, you are able to work with a skilled professional who specializes in MarCons. Although I'm not putting it in a precise manner, you'll receive an antibiotic spray, known as BEG spray. I went with a more natural method using a mixture of salt, water, tri-salts and xylitol.

Dr. Deitrich Klinghardt has a Formula Using:

*4 cups of H2O that is tepid (not overly hot and and not too cold)

*1 tablespoon Himalayan salt

1.25 tablespoons Kal brand xylitol, as this is an extremely fine powder alternatively, use any other brand.

1.25 tablespoons Tri-salts (he makes use of baking soda)

In a glass jar, shake the ingredients listed above until the mixture has dissolved. Keep the mixture for use later.

I utilize the SinuPulse Elite to flush out my sinuses by using the Dr. Klinghardt's formula. It's an sophisticated Nasal Sinus Irrigation System recommended by top pediatricians, allergists, and ENTs. It was developed and manufactured in Switzerland. It's a pulsatile device. The smooth, gentle pulsing of the solution with a custom tip is a way to cleanse the sinuses and nose free of dust, allergens pollen and dirt, and actually aids in enhancing the flow of ciliary blood.

SinuPulse Elite is a great option for sinus problems. SinuPulse Elite is beneficial for nasal snoring that is caused by sinuses as well as environmental conditions such as smoke, pollution, smog or chemical exposure. It is recommended by Dr. Robert Iver, author of the best-selling book "Sinus Survival," wrote, "I recommend the SinuPulse as the best modern irrigation device, as well as the one that is capable of providing a moisturizing mist spray, and more treatments that completely eliminate sinus infections or treating sinusitis. It is able to help fast and significantly. "

I bought mine from Amazon.com. I was able to test MarCons negative after 2 years of using the Dr. Klinghardt's formula, and also employing SinuPulse Elite. It's amazing! It's also the reason I stayed away from antibiotics. I know that some people make use of neti pots. I would not recommend them.

MarCons as well as other infections can occur if a patient suffers from a deviated septum. There are times when you notice a nose that is crooked. If you aren't sure if you're suffering from a deviated septum consult your doctor. If the problem isn't corrected through surgery, the above nasal wash must be used regularly.

The Nasopure nasal wash bottle can be an cost-effective way to wash out your sinuses. It can also be carried on a trip. It is made by people with disabilities who are adults. It is BPA free, manufactured in Missouri as well as being USA and FDA certified. It is available for purchase at Walgreens.

Third Pearl - Tudca

A few years ago, I was able to meet an athlete using steroids. Did you realize that the enzymes in his liver were elevated due to steroids? AL, -alamine transanudase +AST - aspartate Transaminase are liver enzymes along with other organs of the body.

He would then take an ingredient called Tudca to reduce the enzyme level to stay on steroids. Tudca proved effective and is recognized by bodybuilders.

For the person who is chronically sick the liver enzymes tend to be excessive. I was able to meet a young teen in the Dallas

Environmental Health Center who had elevated liver enzymes which did not go down despite treatment. Her mother stayed in my house one evening and asked me to suggest how her daughter could go about completing an enema with coffee.

If it were the day today I would have advised Tudca immediately. However the coffee enema was successful in achieving the purpose of decreasing her liver enzyme levels.

Fourth Pearl - Hormetic Stress

I've heard the term"hormetic" stress being that is used to treat chronic diseases. Hormetic stress occurs when you apply a positive source of stress on the body to cause it to grow more resilient. The examples in this book include sauna, ozone sauna the colon cleanse and coffee-based enemas LED Zyto or Asyra treatments mini-trampoline as well as antioxidants. I recommend anyone suffering from adrenal fatigue or chronic fatigue to take these treatment options. The two conditions are both present in a variety of areas.

If someone who is chronically sick utilizes cold water following the shower, it will help your adrenal glands. This may seem counterintuitive however it is effective. When I first heard about the benefits of cold in helping my recovery, I yelled at my friend and said, "My adrenal glands have enough stress." He was kind enough to suggest that I do it for 30 seconds. I'm still doing it now... just a bit longer! Aerobic workouts that are hard to train in can be a great hormetic stress for healthy individuals but wouldn't be a good choice for chronically ill patients.

Additionally, the concept of using a low dose exposure to chemicals for people with MCS would be an unhealthy hormetic strain. It's not working. Therefore, hormetic stress is not a form of exercise or eating a healthy diet could be done for those who are chronically ill too. In case you are unable to jump on the mini-trampolinethen have someone else jump for you while you are sitting on it. It's just as efficient, particularly if you are sitting in a wheelchair. When I was extremely sick, my friend gave me a mini trampoline. I ran for about 20 minutes and vomited for eight hours. It was enough emotional stress. I could not see a trampoline in months. I hated it. Five minutes of time would suffice. Every person has their individual level of hormetic stress. It's a balance. If you exercise lightly and get sick over two weeks, it's a sign of hormonal stress. If you are a chronically sick person, it might be a good thing. It is possible to find the equilibrium of positive and negative hormetic stress.

Fifth Pearl - Naltrexone

Naltrexone is a substance utilized in the treatment of addiction. It is prescribed for 150mgs. It is being used to treat chronically ill patients at 4.5mgs. It's an immuno booster. Your doctor will provide you with a prescription along with instructions. Naltrexone was a huge help in the reduction of my sensitivities to chemical. I took it off for a month, then recommenced as I was becoming chemically sensitive. Today, I'm on 4.5mgs of the drug naltrexone.

Chapter 21: Food & Hypothyroidism

Hypothyroidism is a complex medical condition that is difficult to treat. In reality, anything related to your lifestyle and diet could negatively impact the treatment. Certain foods can stimulate the thyroid gland, other foods may slow it down.

While some foods may increase the metabolism of your body, other foods stop your hormones from getting absorption. Even with all of these issues, you is able to live in the absence of hypothyroidism by having the proper understanding of nutrition and food. This chapter is about that!

Foods that can aggravate hypothyroidism

Here's a list with a few foods which you should stay clear of at all cost. These foods have been known to cause problems with treatment for hypothyroidism and should be avoided if wish to cure the thyroid issue.

Brassica veggies: Brassica vegetables or cruciferous vegetables have been known to affect your thyroid hormones in the body. If your body is digesting these foods, your thyroid gland is unable to absorb iodine, and the lack of iodine leads to decreased function that the thyroid gland. So, you should limit or eliminate the consumption (5 1 ounce per day) of kale, cabbage turnip, broccoli, as well as the cauliflower (all comprising brassicas).

Soy products: Soy-based products contain plant-based phytoestrogen, which has been proven to affect your body's capacity to utilize thyroid hormones. Furthermore, research has concluded that foods containing soy increase the risk of developing hypothyroidism. As a precaution, you should reduce the amount of soy you consume or, in the event that you can, eliminate soy-based products.

Sugar: As you've probably guessed already, hypothyroidism is a condition that will eventually slow the metabolism of your body. This means that you'll increase your weight faster, and the levels of bad cholesterol will increase. Therefore, nutritionists advise to stay clear of sugar consumption. Sugar-rich food are loaded with empty calories , which means that you are getting lower amounts of fiber, nutrients or vitamins in the large quantity of calories consumed. For example, a piece of cake can contain as much as 500 calories! However, break it down into the nutritional value of the cake and you'll discover little to none of the vitamins, minerals or fiber in any way.

Gluten: Gluten could affect the lining of your stomach, which can reduce your absorption rate of thyroid hormone replacement medicines. Constipation is a common occurrence in hypothyroid patients and, therefore, eating whole grain gluten that have higher levels of fiber aids.

Fiber: Since the expression says "too much of anything is bad" Consuming a high levels of fiber may cause health issues in your system. Consuming too much fiber reduces the body's ability to absorb medications employed in thyroid treatment.

Foods that are heavily fried Deep-fried food items such as meat with skin, mayonnaise, as well as fats can block in the absorption and metabolism of thyroid hormones synthetic into the body. Therefore, if you're being treated, doctors advise cutting down on these unhealthy fat food items. Avoid deep-fried food such as butter, margarine, Ghee and heavy pieces of beef. But, it is important to consume fats that are healthy like avocadoes or flax seeds.

Processed food: Foods that are processed contain high amounts of sodium that is detrimental to your body. The general rule is that sodium raises blood pressure, which isn't healthy for your body. When you combine the effects of sodium with the hypothyroidism-related effects (which also raises blood pressure) it becomes dangerous. Therefore, stay away from processed foods.

Alcohol: Alcohol not only reduces the absorption of thyroid hormone but also affects the thyroid gland's capacity to produce sufficient thyroid hormones. It has a negative impact on the gland and interferes with its function. So, it is imperative to stop drinking the alcohol completely in order to ensure that your body is healthy and functioning.

Coffee Consuming coffee while taking thyroid hormone replacement and drinking coffee may affect your body. It could raise your thyroid levels too much. The medications won't be able to stop the hormones that cause this. So, doctors suggest that you take at least 30 minutes before drinking coffee after taking medications.

Foods for hypothyroidism that are hypothyroidism friendly

After giving you a lengthy list of foods that you should not consume, I hope that I didn't break your heart. Whatever the case there's no need to be concerned as your life isn't done. You'll be able to indulge in a variety of delicious food groups and continue taking your thyroid medication. Here's a list of food items that you can consume with a lot of pleasure.

Fish: Fishes such wild salmon or sardines , are rich in Omega 3 fatty acids that lower bad cholesterol and decrease the chances of developing cardiovascular disease. Because hypothyroidism can increase the risk of heart disease A diet that is rich of omega-3 fatty acids could protect you from future issues.

Constipation from whole grains is a typical symptom of hypothyroidism. You can combat it by eating an eating plan that is rich in whole grains. This will boost the amount of fiber you consume and assist in preventing bowel irregularities. Be sure you eat whole grains after taking your medication since they can hinder the absorption of the medication.

Nuts: Nuts are rich in selenium, which aids the thyroid gland to work properly. So, try eating a small amounts of nuts every day. Be careful not to overdo it with nuts since they are high in good fats , however they could increase your weight when consumed in large quantities.

Fruits and vegetables weight gain is a important issue for people suffering from hypothyroidism. eating fresh fruits and vegetables and vegetables, you can ensure you consume fewer calories but also high-density calories will supply your body with the most nutrients with the smallest amount of calories.

Dairy products: A deficiency of vitamin D can be linked to Hashimoto's Disease, that causes hypothyroidism. Therefore, doctors suggest drinking fortified milk that is rich with calcium, vitamin D as well as protein and iodine. To ensure your body is in good shape ensure that you take glasses of milk or consume yogurt every day.

Conclusion

Maintaining a healthy lifestyle isn't easy for the majority of people. If you have more than one thing to do in a single day, which includes caring for your children as well as a job and keeping your marriage in check the situation can become messy and the most important thing to consider is the amount of food you consume. Who would want to keep track of calories when every kid is pestering you about a new toy that they want to purchase, your dog is causing a mess on the floor, and your boss wants to put in some more time every now and then. I felt that I required more than 8 hours during the day, when I was pregnant with my first child. At the time I gave birth to my child number three I could have had an additional 18 hours. I've experienced the discontent that comes over you when you've completed something a thousand times only to have to repeat it again.

But what people do not consider is that the food you consume will affect the way you feel and the amount you complete in a day. It's normal in our carb-driven world to believe, "Ok, I'm tired. Let me take a doughnut break." If this doesn't work you're in need of cookies and a cup of coffee. Then, before you know it is lunch time and a tasty double cheeseburger will be in your soon to come. When the day is over you're exhausted. You've been anything other than tired throughout the day. When does it end?

But, nobody ever considers, "Maybe if I eat this apple, it will keep me focused longer." The food item that fills you up faster that immediately comes to the mind. This is the reason for the aforementioned energy crisis. The solution is described within the book. integrate the above foods into your diet, and you'll feel as though you've been given an extra 8 hours or so per day. This implies that you must replace the bad choices in your food for healthier choices. Many people fall into the trap of assuming of "If I add these healthy foods to the diet I already have, I'll lose weight and feel great."

It's not as easy. If you consume one quarter of 1 teaspoon of pumpkin seeds following having a low-fat muffin you're adding 180 calories to the 250 calories that you consumed through the muffin. The pumpkin seeds are healthy however those from the muffin aren't. Take a bite of pumpkin seeds and half a Cup of cubes from watermelon instead. Make that your sweet fix.

These changes to your diet can be implemented quickly and effectively. Before I started the diet that improved my energy levels and reduced my weight I was adamant that I'd have to commit long hours rearranging everything about my lifestyle to achieve these goals. The mere thought of it made me feel tired and dismotivated. When I began purchasing the right food items and eating them I realized that it doesn't take too any effort or time to choose healthier options. It's all in what that you buy. Be aware of the items you fill your cart with. Did you load that case of Pepsi onto the rung underneath your cart? Did you pick up that box of cookies as well as the frozen strips of chicken? What about swapping the cookies with a bag of apples and throwing away that container of frozen chicken in favour of a container full of fresh chicken breasts?

It doesn't do anyone any favors by filling your fridge and freezer with processed foods. Sure, your kids love it. Manufacturers are careful to include flavor-enhancing chemicals in their food products, to keep your customers returning for more. Who wouldn't be obsessed with potato chips? The delicious, unhealthy fats are waiting to be consumed. Also processed foods can make your life easier, or do they? Yes, you could multitask better if you could simply pop that frozen pizza in the oven rather than slaving over a meal that you cooked at home.

But how much will it actually benefit you to fill yourself up with carbs that are fast acting? What does these empty calories accomplish when they get into the digestive tract? Is it worth feeling exhausted all the time, adding weight to your already exhausted body daily? If so, then you would not have bought this book to begin with.

Mother Nature has blessed us with healthy, tasty food options galore. So why not benefit from this instead? The manufacturers who make the trendy chicken nuggets and sports drinks that you purchase frequently don't have a vested interest in your health. They're not concerned about your weight loss, and your energy level so long as you continue to return to buy more. Mother Nature, however, isn't able to make a profit out of your eating habits. You can either eat the greens blueberries, broccoli, or other greens she gives you or you do not. It's entirely up to you.

You are responsible for your diet. You are responsible for your weight. The best part is that you control your energy levels. You can let yourself be brimming with energy and lose weight enough to fit into that pair of jeans you wore to college. I did it, and I'm happy! It's your turn now. Do you have the ability to control your diet? I'm hoping so. In the meantime I wish you best of luck and good outcomes and I'm hoping you feel a sense of satisfaction from making these little changes to help you become healthier and happier.

www.ingramcontent.com/pod-product-compliance
Lightning Source LLC
Chambersburg PA
CBHW060322030426
42336CB00011B/1163